The Occupational Therapy Student Guide to Understanding Identity

The Occupational Therapy Student Guide to Understanding

IDENTITY

BRIDGING DIFFERENCES AND CREATING COMMUNITIES

**Dr Razan Hamed, Vikram Pagpatan,
and André Johnson**

Jessica Kingsley Publishers
London and Philadelphia

First published in Great Britain in 2026 by Jessica Kingsley Publishers
An imprint of John Murray Press

2

Copyright © Dr Razan Hamed, Vikram Pagpatan, and André Johnson 2026

A CIP catalogue record for this title is available from the
British Library and the Library of Congress

ISBN 978 1 80501 975 6
eISBN 978 1 80501 976 3

Printed and bound in the United States by Integrated Books International

Jessica Kingsley Publishers' policy is to use papers that are natural,
renewable and recyclable products and made from wood grown in
sustainable forests. The logging and manufacturing processes are expected
to conform to the environmental regulations of the country of origin.

Jessica Kingsley Publishers
Carmelite House
50 Victoria Embankment
London EC4Y 0DZ

www.jkp.com

John Murray Press
Part of Hodder & Stoughton Ltd
An Hachette Company

The authorised representative in the EEA is Hachette Ireland, 8 Castlecourt
Centre, Dublin 15, D15 XTP3, Ireland (email: info@hbgi.ie)

Contents

Introduction 9

What is this book about?   9

What is included?   10

How to use this book   11

1. **Diversity, Equity, Inclusion, and Other Aspects of Social
   Justice (DEI+): You, They, and Us** 13

RAZAN HAMED PHD., OTR/L

Chapter overview   13

Introduction   15

Why learn about DEI+?   16

DEI+ and cultural humility   21

Student DEI+ advocacy in education   23

DEI+ in clinical and fieldwork learning   24

Let's think about it   26

References   28

2. **Allyship, Accompliceship, and Advocacy: How Can I Help?** . . . 29

ANDRÉ JOHNSON MS, COTA/L, ROH

Chapter overview   29

Allyship, accompliceship, and advocacy: Why are they important? 31

Allyship   34

Accompliceship   36

Advocacy   38

Allyship, accompliceship, and advocacy on fieldwork   40

Let's think about it   41

References   42

3. **Bias and Microaggressions** 44

RAZAN HAMED PHD., OTR/L

Chapter overview   44

Introduction 46

All things bias 47

Bias and difficult conversations in the classroom 50

Bias and intersectionality 53

Let's think about it 57

References 59

4. **Privilege and Critical Consciousness** 61

VIKRAM PAGPATAN EDD., OTR/L, FAOTA

Chapter overview 61

Introduction 63

Critical consciousness: What is it and what does it mean for
students and practitioners? 64

Recognizing factors related to privilege: Are accountability and
ethics included? 70

Let's think about it 73

References 75

5. **Cultural Humility**. 77

RAZAN HAMED PHD., OTR/L

Chapter overview 77

Introduction 79

Cultural humility in the classroom 82

Cultural humility and community engagement 83

Cultural humility in fieldwork education and clinical practice 85

Cultural humility, privilege, and intersectionality 87

Let's think about it 90

References 92

6. **Empathy and Professionalism** 93

VIKRAM PAGPATAN EDD, OTR/L, FAOTA

Chapter overview 93

Introduction 95

Empathy, sympathy, and clinical empathy 96

Empathy, professionalism, and e-professionalism 101

Empathy and accountability, and digital citizenship 101

Let's think about it 107

References 108

7. **Fieldwork and Capstone: Stay Quiet, It's Fieldwork** 110

ANDRÉ JOHNSON MS, COTA/L, ROH

Chapter overview 110

Fieldwork: The journey, experience, and entry into the profession   112
DEI+ in fieldwork   118
Navigating tough FW situations and de-escalation on fieldwork   120
Fieldwork coordinators and educators   122
Fieldwork education and difficult conversations in the classroom   124
Let's think about it   125
References   126

8. **Student to Clinician**   128
RAZAN HAMED PHD., OTR/L AND VIKRAM PAGPATAN EDD., OTR/L, FAOTA
Chapter overview   128
From the classroom to the clinic   130
Transition versus transformation   132
The larger picture   133
Professional development, engagement, and DEI+   134
The first year as an occupational therapy practitioner   136
DEI+, allies, advocates, and accomplices, and culture change:
How does the journey continue?   138
DEI+ and the next generations of occupational therapy students   141
Let's think about it   143
References   145

Appendix 1: Characters Across the Book Chapters   147

Appendix 2: Character Matrix   148

About the Authors   154

DEI+ Workbook: Structured Exercises and Discussion Prompts . . .   156
How to use this workbook   156

Index   169

Introduction

Students come to occupational therapy (OT) with raw personal experiences and limited knowledge about the profession or clinical practice in the field. The journey they take during their OT school introduces them to the world of OT as an arena for clinical practice, professional growth, advocacy, leadership, research, and social justice. Like any journey, our experience is shaped by who we are as people, including the intertwined layers of our race, age, gender, ethnicity, faith, ability, sexual orientation, and neurodiversity. This book attempts to shed light on what the journey may look like for students of different folds of diversity. Although this is a book about diverse experiences in OT education, it is nearly impossible to cover all faces of diversity in one book. Therefore, if you do not relate to any of the content described in this book, please let us know so we can address the gap in future writings.

What is this book about?

This book is written for occupational therapy students on issues related to diversity, equity, inclusion, justice, belonging, access, and other aspects of social justice in our communities (DEI+). The book uses a storytelling approach of two students starting a graduate occupational therapy program at college. These two students, Allie and Gemma, are the main characters who represent two distinct racial-ethnic groups, privileges, abilities, and intersectionalities. Although the characters used in this book are fictitious, their experiences may resemble the education and practice of many members of OT communities. Snapshots of their journey (and others in the classroom) are threaded throughout the book using detailed case studies. The book is meant for students to reflect, critically analyze, and discuss how DEI+ affects their education and future practice. The book can be used as an educational textbook for the content and case studies and as material for discussions and conversations about DEI+ in the profession. Students can use the practical strategies threaded throughout the book in their classrooms, didactic and fieldwork experiences, as well as in the transition to clinician roles. The book can also be used as material to create workshops, in-service sessions, and cultural humility training for student-run organizations in the profession.

Although the book is written for occupational therapy students, it can be used by other students in the healthcare fields, such as physical therapy, nursing, speech therapy, physician assistants, and other allied health sectors.

What is included?

The book includes several case studies that use fictitious characters to spotlight different DEI+ aspects, conflicts, and realities inspired by real student experiences. The characters are used as a contrast between two journeys shaped by issues related to DEI+ in modern society. Each chapter starts with a snapshot of students' experiences during OT school and offers other case studies on the topics discussed therein. The case studies are meant to provide relatable, personal, and diverse stories and voices of occupational therapy (OT), occupational therapy assistant (OTA), and doctor of occupational therapy (OTD) students. The stories span the entire OT learning journey, starting from orientation and ending with the first job in clinical practice.

The companion workbook at the end of this volume invites readers to actively apply and internalize the concepts explored throughout the textbook. Through interactive case scenarios, reflective exercises, role plays, and structured debates, the workbook offers an engaging space for translating insight into practice. Designed with students and early-career practitioners in mind, these activities aim to deepen critical thinking, foster cultural humility, and cultivate the skills necessary for equity-centered practice. The goal is to transform learning into lived competence that endures across clinical and professional contexts.

Trigger warning: while you read the content of this book, please be advised that case studies, scenarios, suggested readings, and images may be triggering to some readers given their personal and historical experiences and intersectionality. We recommend seeking support from colleagues or mentors if content may be triggering or upsetting.

How to use this book

- **Opening images:** Each chapter starts with an image that is meant to set the stage from a present or historical context. The images are also meant to highlight the diversity of perspectives in our learning journeys as each student may use that image to approach the content differently.

- **Content and storylines:** The chapters begin with an overview of the content discussed in that section of the book and the characters within that chapter. The chapters preface with a storyline snapshot that acts as a timestamp in the OT journey. We hope that these snapshots in time make it easier for students to follow the storyline that describes DEI+ issues commonly experienced by students at that stage of learning. Each chapter lists the characters used in the case studies therein. Before reading the chapters, we suggest taking a look at the characters included in that chapter by reviewing the character matrix (see Appendix 2). Understanding a character's diverse traits may help you reflect on the DEI+ aspects promoted in the case studies in that chapter.

- **Case studies** and reflective questions are meant to spotlight specific behaviors, actions, and statements that can be problematic for learning or may undermine students' well-being. The reflective pauses are meant to provide students with opportunities to process feelings and thoughts on the case studies and the challenges and solutions they provide. A commentary following each case study is provided to facilitate discussions and shed light on the aspects of DEI+ being discussed. The commentaries also provide suggested actions for the students to take or consider when facing a similar scenario. It is important to remember that these suggestions may or may not apply to all students or all situations, given the nuances of interpersonal interactions and conflicts encountered. Students are encouraged to use these case studies as pauses for thinking and reflection that may inspire effective solutions to their own learning spaces.

- The **"Let's think about it"** sections expand on a case study or a topic with further questions for reflection. To educators adopting the book: the "Let's think about it" sections can be used for small-group discussions, exercises, or student panels. The **"Hot take"** question at the end of each chapter is meant for a deeper reflection on issues that are perceived as delicate, controversial, or difficult to discuss. For each of these "Hot take" questions, one scholastic article is suggested that can help facilitate discussions. These questions are meant as thought-provoking reflections on the wider DEI+ issues in the OT education and community. These can be used for student panel discussions, anonymous polling, or small-group conversations. Additionally, this section can be used for student-run advocacy groups to hold small events or panel discussions.

CHAPTER 1

Diversity, Equity, Inclusion, and Other Aspects of Social Justice (DEI+)

YOU, THEY, AND US

Allie and Gemma meet at orientation

Razan Hamed PhD., OTR/L

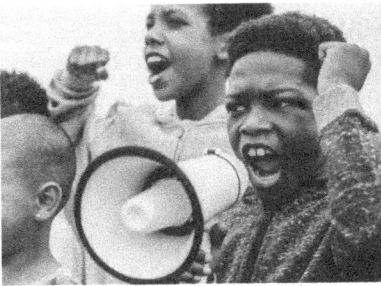

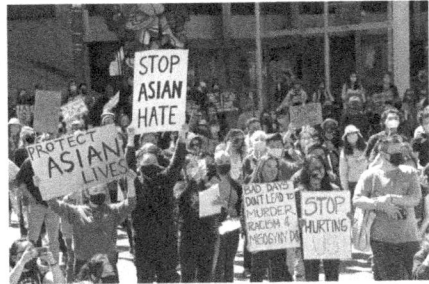

Chapter overview

This chapter introduces students to diversity, equity, inclusion, and justice in occupational therapy education and practice. We discuss the significance of these concepts and their impact on students' academic well-being, mental health, and professional growth. We provide real-life examples of DEI+ challenges in classrooms, fieldwork, and other educational spaces. The chapter lays the groundwork for subsequent chapters in the book, which offer practical strategies and tools to address issues of DEI+ while in the student role. Students are invited to reflect on their understanding of DEI+ concepts and cultural humility throughout the chapter.

Content

- Why learn about DEI+? Case example 1.1: Student diversity—Allie and Gemma meet Dr. Boyle at orientation.
- DEI+ and cultural humility, Case example 1.2: Cultural humility—Allie and Gemma talk about Amihan.
- Student DEI+ advocacy in education, Case example 1.3: Julian talks to the Coalition of Occupational Therapy Advocates for Diversity (COTAD).
- DEI+ in clinical and fieldwork, Case example 1.4: Allie and Gemma meet Israa.
- Let's think about it.

Objectives

1. Understand the need to learn about issues related to DEI+ in the academic and clinical environments of occupational therapy.
2. Recognize basic constructs and terminology related to DEI+.
3. Explore practical strategies for navigating daily experiences and environments, and advocating for inclusive and culturally informed teaching.

Storyline snapshot

Allie and Gemma meet at the orientation event at the Master of Science in Occupational Therapy (MSOT) program at a big university in New York. Gemma identifies as Latino-Black, and Allie identifies as White. The two students start chatting to get to know each other; they exchange information about their undergraduate majors, home states, hobbies, pets, and thoughts about what lay ahead in the program. The two students will take the same classes, work on the same assignments, interact with the same instructors, and complete the same fieldwork requirements. The academic experiences of the two students, albeit identical, are far from similar. Their perspectives reflect the reality of thousands of occupational therapy students. In this book, stories and scenarios experienced by the two students (and others) are described to help the reader envision what it is like to be Gemma or Allie, reflect on their perspectives, and expand their understanding of diversity, equity, inclusion, justice, belonging, and accessibility in occupational therapy.

Characters in this chapter (see the character matrix in Appendix 2 for details)

- Allie and Gemma
- Dr. Boyle
- Memona
- Amihan
- Julian
- Israa

Introduction

If you're Black and don't see yourself in the pages of a book, it makes you put it down.

VILLAROSA, 2022, P.15

The quote by Professor Villarosa threads the concepts of diversity, equity, inclusion, belonging, and representation in one sentence that screams the loud sentiment: diversity matters (Villarosa, 2022). The quote speaks to the reality of many students, practitioners, and educators in occupational therapy. Black, African American, Indigenous, Middle Eastern, Hispanic, Asian, disabled, lesbian, gay, bisexual, transgender, queer, intersex, asexual (LGBTQIA+) people, Jews, Muslims, Sikhs, Buddhists, and so many others from diverse backgrounds are rarely the feature case study in a textbook, the leaders in prominent roles, or the well-represented demographic in any OT program. They are, in a sense, invisible in a predominantly White profession. Underrepresentation can affect students' educational, clinical, or professional experiences and can be demotivating and isolating for students from neglected or marginalized groups or backgrounds. Underrepresentation can also be discouraging for allies or advocates (e.g. students who identify with the majority group) for social justice in their future profession. After all, diversity matters to everyone!

The need to address diversity, equity, and inclusion is not new to occupational therapy or other healthcare professions (Brown *et al.*, 2021; Taff & Blash, 2017; Wilbur *et al.*, 2020). But this book brings it into the spotlight, with practical and useful strategies for all occupational therapy students (minority, majority, and all in between). We aim to promote a mindset that embraces diversity, deconstructs bias and microaggressions, and rejects the status quo around DEI+ in occupational therapy education and the workforce. The content in this book is based on the multifaceted experiences in occupational therapy of educators, practitioners, and researchers. This book is also informed by literature on DEI+ in occupational therapy. A deeper exploration of the research-based literature is recommended while navigating this textbook.

Why learn about DEI+?

Diversity, equity, inclusion, justice, belonging, accessibility, and other aspects of social justice (DEI+) are key elements for a supportive community of occupational therapy practitioners. Diversity is defined as the variations in human-related traits such as age, race, gender identity, ethnicity, ability status, sexual orientation, body size, neurocognitive function, socioeconomic status, and other defining categories. Equity is having fair access to opportunities across various areas of life that will optimize an individual's potential. Inclusion is intentionally involving individuals from different groups in relevant daily matters. Justice is dismantling systemic barriers to resources so that every individual has the opportunity to fulfill their potential. Belonging is the sense of being naturally and deservedly associated with a certain group, community, or context. Accessibility is providing necessary facilitators or accommodations for individuals with restricted abilities to perform daily activities.

Therefore, the American Occupational Therapy Association (AOTA) revised its 2025 vision (from 2017) to emphasize the need for an inclusive profession that serves persons, groups, and populations with equity while considering all aspects of culture and contexts (AOTA, 2020a). The AOTA code of ethics calls for practitioners to treat their clients with justice, fairness, and empathy. Occupational therapy practitioners and educators pride themselves in being empathetic healthcare professionals who serve the needs of individuals, groups, and populations. Yet, we stumble on the need to talk about bias and DEI+ in educational, clinical, and professional contexts in occupational therapy every day. Such conversations are difficult and often avoided by OT stakeholders for several reasons, including the complex and multifaceted nature of these constructs, the lack of education or training on DEI+ matters in OT practice, and the discomfort that accompanies such discussions.

For many occupational therapy and occupational therapy assistants (OTA) students, daily classroom interactions, fieldwork placements, institutional events, advising, and campus life are enriching academic and professional experiences. But for some, these experiences can be uncomfortable, discouraging, or even traumatic experiences that are tainted with microaggressions, implicit bias, and bouts of imposter syndrome (Salvant *et al.*, 2021). Equipping OT/OTA students with tangible tools to address these DEI+ issues in education and practice is one way to move toward an inclusive profession (American Occupational Therapy Association, 2020b, 2020c). Students need to learn about DEI+ not only because they may be experiencing daily micro-traumas first hand (e.g. microaggressions) but because it is consistent with the profession's core values and principles described in the code of ethics.

Experiencing these micro-traumas can affect students' well-being and mental health, which may stunt learning and professional growth. For example, affected students can show resentment and anger (Sue *et al.*, 2007), anxiety, depression, and even post-traumatic stress disorder (Nadal *et al.*, 2019). Students who go through these negative experiences need to be aware of these DEI+ issues to address these traumas and advocate for themselves and others. Students who are less susceptible to these experiences (e.g. those who identify with the majority or are of high socio-economic class) must understand what other people go through daily in order to enhance their sense of empathy (see Chapter 6), which in turn promotes inclusive spaces in the classroom, clinic, and other professional contexts.

Table 1.1 summarizes the basic terminology relevant to DEI+. The AOTA develops and regularly updates the culturally appropriate DEI+ terminology.

Table 1.1: Basic terminology in the context of DEI+

Term	Definition	Significance	Example
Diversity	Differences between individuals that can be attributed to race, gender, ethnicity, faith, ability and disability status, sexual orientation, gender identity, culture, and other macro and micro levels of diversity.	Enhances representative engagement, improves communication, reduces bias.	An entry-level OT/OTA program admits cohorts of students of different racial, ethnic, faith, cultural backgrounds, sexual and gender identities and orientations, ability statuses, etc.
Equity	Fair approach to allocating resources and opportunities to individuals to fulfill their potential.	Increases capacity and performance of persons, groups, and populations and reduces societal tension.	Scheduling the midterm exam on two days (instead of one) for students with chronic health conditions that may limit test stamina.
Inclusion	Actively involving individuals from different groups and backgrounds.	Creates safe spaces that foster a sense of belonging.	Including students of diverse learning abilities in curriculum committees in an OT/OTA program to provide a student's perspective on the learning process.
Justice	Dismantling barriers to resources, including bias, oppression, and privilege.	Meets the needs of individuals and creates a fair experience for everyone.	Revising OT/OTA admission processes and applications to offer applicants the opportunity to explain how racial trauma affected their grades in undergraduate education or access to college preparatory resources.
Belonging	The feeling of being naturally associated with a group, community, or context.	Makes a positive impact on one's relationship in various physical, social, and cultural contexts.	Feeling comfortable in an OT/OTA program because you share common traits with other students (i.e. not feeling isolated).
Accessibility	Having facilitated access in all environments to mitigate personal or environmental barriers to opportunities in daily activities.	Provides the support needed for all individuals to fulfill their potential in daily activities.	Creating accessible spaces in didactic and clinical learning courses (e.g. fieldwork rotations) for students with physical or behavioral disabilities.

Explicit bias	Irrational assumptions or misconceptions about someone's abilities or worth.	Misjudges people's abilities and limits their potential.	Consistently rejecting Hispanic applicants from admission to an OT/OTA program for anticipating their inability to succeed in a rigorous program.
Implicit bias	Unconscious assumptions that stem from associating a group of people with a particular trait. The person inadvertently projects (or acts on) stereotypes, generalizations, or insults without covertly using offensive language.	Perpetuates explicit bias and affects people's mental health.	An instructor assumes that Black students in the classroom would be interested in tutoring support offered by the OT/OTA program.
Cultural humility	Continuous learning about diverse cultures and backgrounds while recognizing the privilege and power associated with, or perceived about, some groups over others.	Encourages an open and reflective mindset about others' lived experiences.	Recognizing the lack of cultural humility of an instructor when discussing the prevalence of chronic conditions in Black or African Americans without discussing the context of access to healthcare (i.e. justice issues) or health literacy (i.e. equity issues).

Note: The terminology used in the DEI+ arena is continuously evolving. New terms emerge to reflect new realities; some are modified, rephrased, or changed; and others are retired for being irrelevant or limited in scope. At the time of writing this book, this is some of the essential terminology students and future practitioners must be familiar with to embrace DEI+ practice.

CASE EXAMPLE 1.1: Student diversity

During the social part of orientation, the students sit in small groups of five with a faculty member, Dr. Boyle, to become familiar with the program staff. Three students (including Allie) and Dr. Boyle identify as White. The other two students are Gemma, who identifies as Black, and Memona, who identifies as South Asian. Gemma and Memona scan the room trying to find who else looks like them. Allie does not.

Dr. Boyle introduces herself to the students and talks about the courses she teaches in the program and recent research projects. The students introduce themselves and talk about their undergraduate experiences and what they like to do when not studying. When Gemma introduces herself, Dr. Boyle says, "How do you spell your name?"

Gemma answers, and Dr. Boyle responds, "With a G—nice!" Dr. Boyle does not ask anyone else to spell their name. Gemma is confused by the response but "brushes it off" and continues listening to the conversations. When the time is up, students rotate around the room to meet other faculty members as per the schedule. Gemma whispers to herself, "Well, that didn't take long!"

Reflection pause

- How would you describe Dr. Boyle?
- Why do you think Dr. Boyle asks that question to Gemma and not others?
- What do you think Gemma is thinking when she says, "Well, that didn't take long?"

Commentary on Case example 1.1

The question asked by Dr. Boyle, albeit innocuous, signals Gemma out. The fact that she only asks Gemma how to spell her name and does not ask other students about name spells is insensitive, if not discriminatory, at face value. Likely, Dr. Boyle is only curious to know how Gemma's name is spelled, since it could be spelled with a J instead. However, we need to be mindful of how our questions can come across to other people no matter what the original intent is from that question. Spelling variations in the Black community have various historical annotations (such as the segregation era, slavery, and the development of Black culture). This history must be respected and considered in conversations about names, their spellings, and meanings. Faculty members need to be mindful of such history as they may trigger a feeling of loneliness or intergenerational racial trauma in Black students.

A more mindful way to handle that interaction with Dr. Boyle is to explain why she asked the question. For example, she could say, "I know other Gemmas with a J, so I am just curious." The lack of this explanation may lead Gemma to think that being Black is the reason for that question, given that Black names can have spelling variations to common European or biblical names (Cook *et al.*, 2022).

Gemma could also voice her concern (if any) with that question by following up with a clarification, "I am just curious what you think it spelled like," or, "Do you know many Gemmas?"

DEI+ and cultural humility

DEI+ is the building block of cultural humility in clinical practice. Cultural humility is the intentional and ongoing learning about diverse cultures and backgrounds while recognizing the privilege and power associated with or perceived about some groups over others (Tervalon & Murray-García, 1998). Understanding the diverse continuum of function (e.g. ability status) in different contexts (e.g. physical, social, and cultural environments) expands the students' perceptions of how others function within different roles and across different occupations. It is that lifelong learning about diverse populations (i.e. diversity), challenges to equitable resources (i.e. equity), exploring interventions to enhance participation (i.e. inclusion), and advocating for the needs of different clients (i.e. justice) that builds up our bias-free knowledge about others (i.e. humility).

There has been a call for shifting to cultural humility in OT pedagogies to enhance a lifelong learning approach when working with diverse populations (Agner, 2020). Cultural humility is not limited to clinical practice; it is critical for healthy classroom dialogue. Cultural humility requires recognizing knowledge gaps about someone's culture and their intersectionality (i.e. how multiple cultural identities influence daily interactions), whether it is a client, a classmate, a co-worker, a teacher, or a fieldwork supervisor. It also requires having a curious and empathetic mindset when interacting with others. For instance, when you understand how a classmate is triggered by a comment made by an instructor in the classroom, your sense of cultural humility will help identify the triggers and the bias experienced by that person. It also enables you to advocate for yourself or others and address these incidents empathetically. This will lead to a more connected community of occupational therapy students and future practitioners.

CASE EXAMPLE 1.2: Cultural humility in the classroom

Gemma and Allie are discussing an interaction that happened in class with their peer Amihan, who identifies as Filipino American. The interaction occurs during a class about dysphasia and swallowing disorders in older adults. The instructor describes the OT feeding approach in choking incidents in older adults. The instructor comments, "Certain food textures may be more hazardous than others, such as greasy Chinese food or dumplings, for example." The instructor then looks at Amihan and says, "I've honestly never tried Chinese food. You look as if you would know a good example, Amihan! Can you think of a popular food item from your culture that can pose a choking hazard in that population and explain why?" Amihan smiles and shakes her head without providing an answer. The instructor smiles back and moves on with the class.

Reflection pause

- What do you think Amihan is thinking about at that moment?
- What would you say to Amihan after class?
- Do you think this interaction could affect Amihan's mental health? Explain how or why not.
- If you relate to this incident, describe how you would react to the instructor's comment.
- Should Gemma or Allie say something to Amihan or the instructor? Explain your answer.
- Why do you think Gemma is upset?

Commentary on Case example 1.2

This example describes a deceivingly innocuous classroom exchange meant to encourage clinical reasoning when thinking about feeding interventions. The instructor's poor phrasing of "greasy Chinese food" is problematic and lacks cultural humility. First, it is generalizing (i.e. extending one's perception of a community to all its members without inspecting perception) and may be perceived as stereotyping or offensive to some students who identify with Chinese descent.

Additionally, the instructor assumes that Amihan is of Chinese heritage based on the her physical appearance. This incident may interfere with the student's learning experience as these microaggressive encounters may affect the student's attention, focus, or clinical reasoning at that moment. The incident can also trigger other students witnessing this exchange as it may resemble similar encounters with the same instructor or others in the program. This classroom moment might be more informative if the student is well-equipped to navigate that dialogue and the instructor is well-informed on cultural humility.

Cultural humility is a lifelong learning process that can take some educators longer to navigate. Students face similar interactions in OT classrooms across the United States daily. Students must be offered classroom experiences that embrace diversity and inclusivity and provide safe learning and professional growth spaces.

Student DEI+ advocacy in education

Students are offered numerous active learning opportunities across different contexts, including classrooms, assignments, labs, fieldwork experiences, simulation labs, community-based settings, service learning trips, and virtual education. These opportunities are expected to provide an immersive learning journey where OT students can develop their clinical reasoning skills, practical skillsets, and professional identity. However, the profession was based on models and theories that are euro-centric, developed by White scholars, or based on Western values on independence and occupation (Hammell, 2013). Therefore, critical appraisal of the OT curricula and education by educators and students is necessary for anti-racist education. Students of all races and backgrounds should advocate for inclusive curricula with DEI+-oriented threads and pillars. Students should be engaged in their education and informed on how curricula are designed in their OT programs.

These are some examples of ways students can engage in the learning process:

- Provide feedback on DEI+ content in the curriculum.
- Request inclusive teaching approaches to instruction.
- Report DEI+ issues in instructor and classroom communication.
- Advocate for opportunities to provide identified or anonymous feedback on DEI+ issues around the classroom experience.
- Form student-led organizations within the program to address DEI+ issues in the educational environment.

CASE EXAMPLE 1.3: Advocacy in OT education

The occupational therapy assistant program at University X has just established its Coalition of Occupational Therapy Advocates for Diversity (COTAD) chapter. Julian, an occupational therapy assistant student who identifies as a Hispanic male, reaches out to the chapter leadership to express his concerns about a particular instructor who keeps referring to non-documented immigrants as "Mexicans."

Julian has a physical disability that means he uses a cane to walk independently. He has concerns about the accessibility of the classroom, with limited space to maneuver in the lab space. Julian hesitates to share his concern with the instructor, advisor, or program director, all of whom identify as White, able-bodied females. He feels that his concerns may not sound like a "big deal" to others. The COTAD leaders reach out to the program director to explore the possibility of establishing an anonymous reporting system that can be used with students who prefer to remain anonymous when reporting academic concerns. The program director schedules a meeting with COTAD to explore options for communicating similar situations in the future.

Reflection pause

- What is the difference between Mexicans and Hispanics?
- What do you think is the power of a student-led organization in student advocacy?

Commentary on Case example 1.3

This scenario describes a trust issue many students can experience in the classroom. An established student-led organization can form a communication channel between the program and the students. Additionally, a student-led organization can empower some students who feel uncomfortable in any of the advocacy activities mentioned above.

DEI+ in clinical and fieldwork learning

Starting fieldwork education can be an exciting time for many OT students. However, for some students, the experience can be overwhelming and traumatizing. For example, students with diverse mental and physical health conditions (e.g. anxiety, trauma, medical conditions), diverse socioeconomic status (e.g. limited independent transportation), diverse learning abilities (e.g. receive learning accommodations), or diverse faith and religious backgrounds (e.g. Hindu, orthodox Jewish) may have specific needs to be addressed when assigned fieldwork placements. Students must receive equitable and fair fieldwork assignments that consider their needs and provide just and reasonable accommodations.

Implicit and explicit bias is evident in occupational therapy professionals (Abou-Arab & Mendonca, 2021). Implicit bias is unconscious misjudgments that stem from associating a group of people with a particular trait (Boylewald & Banaji, 1995; Holroyd *et al.*, 2017). Explicit bias is overtly expressed prejudice based on faulty conceptions of a group of people (Boylewald & Krieger, 2006)). Implicit bias is more common in higher education than explicit bias, where people inadvertently project stereotypes, generalizations, or insults without covertly using offensive language. Therefore, one of the challenges students must be prepared for is working with biased or under-informed fieldwork supervisors. Consider the interaction between a student and a fieldwork supervisor in a mental health setting in Case example 1.4.

CASE EXAMPLE 1.4: Implicit bias and stereotypes

During the "Meet the seniors" part of orientation, the incoming students talk to the older cohort in the OT program about their clinical education experience. Gemma and Allie are talking to Israa about fieldwork rotations. Israa identifies as a Muslim cisgender woman. She describes the practice setting where she completed Fieldwork II, including the site placement process, and what she liked and disliked most in her experience. She ends by saying, "Good luck to you both, and Gemma, if you have questions about dealing with 'difficult' supervisors, let me know." Allie responds humorously, "Hey, I may have questions too!" Israa then says, "Oh trust me, you will be fine, girl!" Allie smiles and responds, "I hope so." Gemma smiles at the conversations, but she seems uncomfortable.

Reflection pause

- What do you think of Israa's comments to Gemma?
- What do you feel about Israa's statement to Allie?
- Why do you think Gemma looks uncomfortable?

Commentary on Case example 1.4

This scenario describes a common interaction between new and older students in many OT and OTA programs. Given the stressful nature of fieldwork experiences, students tend to exchange information about fieldwork and helpful tips to navigate this critical milestone. Bias incivility, and even bullying may exist in fieldwork education. Students, especially those from marginalized groups, may experience bias and discrimination by fieldwork supervisors, peers, and even clients. Israa is alluding to potential prejudice and discrimination that Gemma may face because she is Black. Although Allie may also experience bias and discrimination during fieldwork education, Israa implies that it may not be the same kind of bias that Gemma may experience. Some students may find that "heads up" helpful, but others may find it isolating and uncomfortable, as Gemma does.

Let's think about it

A few weeks after orientation, Gemma runs into Israa, whom she met at orientation. They casually greet each other and exchange a few check-in questions. Gemma asks Israa about their interaction at orientation, "Can I ask you a question? What did you mean by your comment about 'difficult' supervisors back at orientation? Israa smiles and shares the following experience: when Israa was completing her fifth week into Level II fieldwork in an inpatient behavioral health facility, she worked with a client diagnosed with schizophrenia on oral hygiene as a self-care activity. While breaking down the activity into smaller steps, the client looked at her and said, "Why are you covering your hair?" Israa responded, "Oh! It is a personal preference and for religious reasons." The client nodded his head and followed up with a couple of questions. Israa answered the questions briefly and then redirected the client to the activity. While debriefing with the fieldwork supervisor, Israa mentioned the exchange that took place earlier with the client about her head covering. The supervisor nodded her head and provided the following feedback, "I think you handled the situation well by redirecting the client to the activity. I recommend that next time you don't entertain questions from clients about personal matters like this; it can be tricky when you wear something that makes you stand out in a place like this. I understand that it's your religion, but you must be careful with these conversations; you're lucky if none of these people think you're a terrorist or something. Don't worry. I am not going to mention this in your midterm evaluation."

Recap

This scenario describes a critical time in fieldwork education: midterm evaluation. It can be a stressful checkpoint for many students. The fieldwork supervisor did not handle the conversation with the students with cultural humility. The supervisor should check in with the students on how they feel after this exchange and offer support if needed. Instead, the supervisor made microaggressive comments when she said, "When you wear something that makes you stand out." This could have affected the student's performance in that fieldwork rotation and can affect her mental health.

Reflective thinking

- How do you think this interaction affected Israa's mental health during or after the exchange with the client and fieldwork supervisor?

Critical thinking

- Think of an appropriate response by Israa to the supervisor's comments about her religion and head scarf.

Action-oriented thinking

- Think of one action Israa can take in the *classroom* to address this experience (e.g. address this issue in a classroom conversation).
- Think of one action Israa can take at the program level to address this experience (e.g. talk to the academic fieldwork coordinator)

HOT TAKE

Occupational therapy is a healthcare profession, not a social justice profession. It is not our job to fix social inequalities. Does it matter that we learn about DEI+?

Suggested reading to navigate this question: "Promoting justice, diversity, equity, and inclusion through caring communities: Why it matters to occupational therapy" (Suarez-Balcazar *et al.*, 2023).

References

Abou-Arab, A., & Mendonca, R. (2021). Exploring implicit and explicit racial bias in OT professionals. *American Journal of Occupational Therapy, 75*(2), 7512500020p1–7512500020p1. https://doi.org/10.5014/ajot.2021.75S2-PO20

Agner, J. (2020). Moving from cultural competence to cultural humility in occupational therapy: A paradigm shift. *American Journal of Occupational Therapy, 74*(4), 7404347010p1–7404347010p7. https://doi.org/10.5014/ajot.2020.038067

American Occupational Therapy Association. (2020a). Occupational therapy's commitment to diversity, equity, and inclusion. *American Journal of Occupational Therapy, 74*(3), 7413410030p1–7413410030p6. https://doi.org/10.5014/ajot.2020.74S3002

American Occupational Therapy Association. (2020b). Educator's guide for addressing cultural awareness, humility, and dexterity in occupational therapy curricula. *American Journal of Occupational Therapy, 74*(3), 7413420003p1–7413420003p19. https://doi.org/10.5014/ajot.2020.74S3005

American Occupational Therapy Association. (2020c). Occupational Therapy Code of Ethics. *American Journal of Occupational Therapy, 74*(3), 7413410005p1–7413410005p13. https://doi.org/10.5014/ajot.2020.74S3006

Brown, K., Lamont, A., Do, A., & Schoessow, K. (2021). Increasing racial and ethnic diversity in occupational therapy education: The role of Accreditation Council for Occupational Therapy Education (ACOTE®) Standards. *American Journal of Occupational Therapy, 75*(3), 7503347020. https://doi.org/10.5014/ajot.2021.047746

Cook, L. D., Parman, J., & Logan, T. (2022). The antebellum roots of distinctively black names. *Historical Methods: A Journal of Quantitative and Interdisciplinary History, 55*(1), 1–11. https://doi.org/10.1080/01615440.2021.1893877

Boylewald, A. G. & Banaji, M. R. (1995). Implicit social cognition: Attitudes, self-esteem, and stereotypes. *Psychological Review, 102*(1), 4–27. https://doi.org/10.1037/0033-295X.102.1.4

Boylewald, A. G. & Krieger, L. H. (2006). Implicit bias: Scientific foundations. *California Law Review, 94*(4), 945. https://doi.org/10.2307/20439056

Hammell, K. R. (2013). Occupation, well-being, and culture: Theory and cultural humility. *Canadian Journal of Occupational Therapy, 80*(4), 224–234. doi: 10.1177/0008417413500465

Holroyd, J., Scaife, R., & Stafford, T. (2017). What is implicit bias? *Philosophy Compass, 12*(10), e12437. https://doi.org/10.1111/phc3.12437

Nadal, K. L., Erazo, T., & King, R. (2019). Challenging definitions of psychological trauma: Connecting racial microaggressions and traumatic stress. *Journal for Social Action in Counseling & Psychology, 11*(2), 2–16. https://doi.org/10.33043/JSACP.11.2.2-16

Salvant, S., Kleine, E. A., & Gibbs, V. D. (2021). Be heard—we're listening: Emerging issues and potential solutions from the voices of BIPOC occupational therapy students, practitioners, and educators. *American Journal of Occupational Therapy, 75*(6), 7506347010. https://doi.org/10.5014/ajot.2021.048306

Suarez-Balcazar, Y., Arias, D., & Muñoz, J. P. (2023). Promoting justice, diversity, equity, and inclusion through caring communities: Why it matters to occupational therapy. *American Journal of Occupational Therapy, 77*(6), 7706347020. https://doi.org/10.5014/ajot.2023.050416

Sue, D. W., Capodilupo, C. M., Torino, G. C., Bucceri, J. M., *et al.* (2007). Racial microaggressions in everyday life: Implications for clinical practice. *American Psychologist, 62*(4), 271–286. https://doi.org/10.1037/0003-066X.62.4.271

Taff, S. D. & Blash, D. (2017). Diversity and inclusion in occupational therapy: Where we are, where we must go. *Occupational Therapy in Health Care, 31*(1), 72–83. https://doi.org/10.1080/07380577.2016.1270479

Tervalon, M. & Murray-García , J. (1998). Cultural humility versus cultural competence: A critical distinction in defining physician training outcomes in multicultural education. *Journal of Health Care for the Poor and Underserved, 9*(2), Article 2.

Villarosa, L. (2022). *Under the Skin: Racism, Inequality, and the Health of a Nation.* Scribe Publications.

Wilbur, K., Snyder, C., Essary, A. C., Reddy, S., Will, K. K., & Saxon, M. (2020). Developing workforce diversity in the health professions: A social justice perspective. *Health Professions Education, 6*(2), 222–229. https://doi.org/10.1016/j.hpe.2020.01.002

CHAPTER 2

Allyship, Accompliceship, and Advocacy

"HOW CAN I HELP?"

Cheyenne advocates: "Hair is not a dress code"

André Johnson MS, COTA/L, ROH

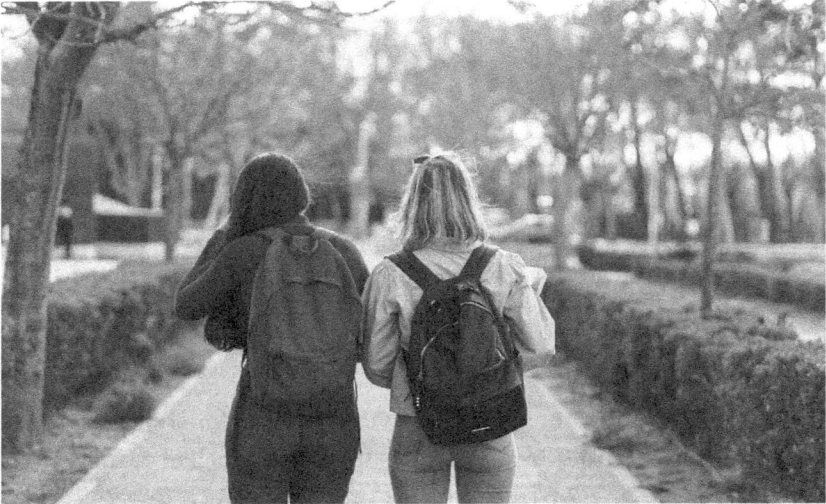

Chapter overview

This chapter introduces the concepts of allyship, accompliceship, and advocacy (AAA) as intricate components of the student experience within occupational therapy education and the professional growth of occupational therapy (OT) and occupational therapy assistant (OTA) students. The chapter reviews the concepts of AAA and their role in creating inclusive classroom spaces, clinical education, and interactions with peers, educators, and clients. We provide community-inspired instances of AAA, and pathways for students and educators to promote cohesive student communities authentically. Students are invited to reflect on their understanding of DEI+ concepts and cultural humility throughout the chapter.

Content

- Allyship, Case example 2.1: Allie and Gemma stand with Dr. Singh in anatomy.
- Accompliceship, Case example 2.2: Cheyenne calls for the creation of a student advisory board.
- Advocacy, Case example 2.3: Amihan runs for AOTA student delegate.
- AAA and fieldwork, Case example 2.4: Malik reports racist remarks by the fieldwork educator.
- Let's think about it.

Objectives

1. Identify the significance of AAA within academic and clinical education.
2. Describe behaviors and acts related to AAA.
3. Apply strategies to become an ally, accomplice, and advocate to address bias and discriminatory learning environments.

Storyline snapshot

The first semester of the OT didactic is usually a time of great transition. Starting a journey in an allied health profession like occupational therapy is never an easy transition, as there is so much to get used to. Not only is there the typical "nervousness" and dynamics of not knowing anyone potentially in play; there is also a vulnerability in opening yourself up to another individual. There is an adjustment to what is considered professional and the expectation of how you should speak, for example. Simply put, there are a lot of changes and adjustments to be made.

In this chapter, Gemma and Allie will dive into typical first-year OT program classes such as anatomy, kinesiology, and introduction to OT. Students during this first semester are introduced to their student occupational therapy association (SOTA) and other leadership and advocacy-oriented actions. Follow the difference faces of allyship and advocacy in the case examples in this chapter.

Characters in this chapter (see character matrix in Appendix 2 for details)

- Allie and Gemma
- Amihan
- Cheyenne[1]
- Malik
- Dr. Campbell
- Dr. Taylor
- Dr. Klein
- Dr. Singh
- Dr. Cruz

Allyship, accompliceship, and advocacy: Why are they important?

When people care for you and cry for you, they can straighten out your soul.

LANGSTON HUGHES

During the first few months of occupational therapy school, students engage in the process of acquainting themselves with one another, discerning not only their identities but also their likes and dislikes. While acquaintances are made by name, a deeper understanding of individuals emerges through familiarity with their personalities and preferences. Although there are instances of shared interests, often disparities arise. Recognizing the necessity for collaborative efforts and mutual support,

---

1   Cheyenne is an ethnicity and Algonquian language, as well as a name. In this book, we use this word as a name.

students acknowledge the imperative of solidarity to excel in their OTA or OT program. Essential concepts such as allyship and accompliceship, encountered in this discourse, are assimilated through interpersonal interactions with peers and faculty, fostering reciprocal relationships. To be clear, allyship and accompliceship are actions, not identities (Cullen *et al.*, 2022).

Moreover, the establishment of rapport with faculty members and peers is paramount, as they play a pivotal role in the educational journey. However, the evaluative aspect of their role may elicit feelings of discomfort or apprehension among students, particularly regarding academic performance. Despite the emphasis on learning over grades, the personal significance attached to one's grade point average (GPA) can engender feelings of inadequacy, especially compared to perceived peer success in academic work.

Amid these academic pressures, achieving equilibrium between academic pursuits and personal well-being poses a formidable challenge. The congruence between individual students, fieldwork educators (FWEs), and the setting environment is instrumental in fostering an educational experience conducive to holistic growth. Moreover, students are entrusted with the responsibility of contributing to the well-being of others, necessitating the acquisition of adept communication skills and the delineation of professional boundaries.

Navigating the intricacies of professional discourse and tone and assimilating constructive feedback are integral components of professional development that require education, time, training, and perseverance (Burgess *et al.*, 2020). Additionally, advocating for oneself within the subordinate role presents a notable challenge, underscoring the significance of self-assertion in the educational landscape.

Despite the trials inherent in this academic pursuit, a robust support system remains indispensable. While geographical distance may separate students from familial and social networks, the shared commitment to their occupational therapy educational program serves as a unifying force. With the tangible goal of attaining the status of occupational therapist or occupational therapist assistant within reach, students should remain steadfast in their pursuit of professional and personal fulfillment.

Table 2.1: Terms related to allyship, accompliceship, and advocacy

Term	Definition	Examples in occupational therapy
Allyship	Refers to individuals and actions taken to collaborate with others to fight injustice and inequity. The fundamental objective of allyship is to provide the support needed to "change policies, practices, and the culture" where the inequity is occurring (American Association of Colleges of Nursing, 2024).	Occupational therapy students advocating for Deferred Action for Childhood Arrivals (DACA) classmates to have equal note-taking services in their native preferred language.
Accompliceship	Encompasses allyship, but goes further by directly challenging the existing conditions and injustices. The individuals do this knowing that their comfort and well-being could be at risk.	Occupational therapy practitioners advocating for the inclusion of underrepresented groups of students in their occupational therapy program and the profession overall (e.g. AOTA publicly restated support for Dr. Lela Llorens as the first and only African American Eleanor Clarke Slagle lectureship in 1969 in New Orleans, where local government contested Dr. Llorens's lectureship).
Advocacy	The act or process of supporting a cause or proposal.	Occupational therapy students and practitioners advocating and successfully having DEI+ interwoven into AOTA Vision 2025 as one of the five pillars in the 2019 revision update.
Mentorship	The influence, guidance, or direction given by a mentor. The mentor has a significant responsibility as they are a role model, trusted person, and confidant, and they provide authentic, constructive feedback.	A seasoned occupational therapy practitioner mentoring an underrepresented Fieldwork II student through their early career in orthopedics with objective feedback and support to assist them in their career goal of becoming a certified hand therapist (CHT) and in navigating their early career ambitions.
Mentee	An individual who is being mentored by a mentor. Mentees should demonstrate intentionality and commitment to their personal and professional growth.	A student, young professional, or mid-career professional seeking insight, objective guidance, and empowerment in professional and career development.

cont.

Term	Definition	Examples in occupational therapy
Code-switching	When an individual from an underrepresented or minority group intentionally adjusts their behavior, verbiage, appearance, and/or expression in a way that fits in with the majority dominant group and structure.	An occupational therapy practitioner or student from an underrepresented group "masking" their authentic feelings on a situation due to a lack of trust in the ability to be authentic (e.g. a Palestinian or Israeli OT or OTA student avoiding discussing the Middle East or their culture due to collective majority feelings at the respective university).
Self-advocacy	The expressed ability to identify one's needs and the ability to speak up for oneself.	Occupational therapy students or practitioners standing up for themselves and what is "right" (e.g. an African American male student advocating for paternity leave or considerations due to their child's illness).
Occupational justice	The "occupational rights to inclusive participation in everyday occupations for all, regardless of age, ability, gender, social class, or other differences," and participation in meaningful occupations are determinants of health and lead to adaptation (Nilsson & Townsend, 2010, p.58).	Occupational therapy practitioners and students advocating for the rights of persons with disabilities to equal and equitable access and quality of education in occupational therapy programs and fieldwork and capstone experiences.

Allyship

Allyship refers to individuals and actions taken to collaborate with others to fight injustice and inequity. An "ally" is active and consistent in their thoughts, words, and actions in working in solidarity with a marginalized or oppressed group. It is important to note that allyship is something that can be learned, and not all "allies" originally started as such. Any person can be or become an ally; all that is required is an open mind and the capacity for self-reflection. Once alliances have been established, allyship is not just about expressing support or sympathy but about actively promoting, advocating, and uplifting marginalized voices (De Souza & Schmader, 2025). True allyship comes with confronting one's privileges and biases and using that awareness to work toward actively dismantling systems of oppression (Arif *et al.*, 2022). Allyship recognizes that marginalized groups are not seeking this alliance for mere companionship, but rather to develop an active partnership in the struggle for equality and justice. In the occupational therapy profession, the multicultural, diversity, and inclusion (MDI) networks are active independent organizations that collectively seek support, allyship, and belonging within the field. The MDI networks consist of various organizations: the Association of Asian Americans and Pacific Islanders in Occupational Therapy (AAPI-OT), the National Black Occupational Therapy Caucus Network for LGBTQIA+ Concerns in Occupational Therapy, the Network of Occupational Therapy Practitioners with Disabilities and Supporters (NOTPD), Occupational Therapy for Native Americans (OTNA), Orthodox Jewish Occupational Therapy Chavrusa (OJOTC), and Terapia Ocupacional para Diversidad, Oportunidad, y Solidaridad (TODOS), a network of Hispanic practitioners. These MDI networks represent diverse historically marginalized communities and underrepresented groups. The MDI networks actively seek and offer allyship in support of the diversity of our profession (American Occupational Therapy Association, 2024). Other independent advocacy groups also exist, such as the Arab American Occupational Therapy Group, Brothas in OT, and the BroOT movement.

CASE EXAMPLE 2.1: Allie and Gemma stand with Dr. Singh in anatomy

During the anatomy lab session, Dr. Singh talks about respecting the body from a scientific, spiritual, and ethical lens as the individual donates their body to science and discovery. Dr. Singh allows the group of students to break into seven groups and start the dissection process. Dr. Singh notices one group of students who seem to chat, laugh, and talk while working at their cadaver station. The students are disrespectful of the dissection process, leaving dissected parts uncovered and whispering to each other, "Relax Dr. Shing, they are dead, who cares what we do?" The students ignore Dr. Singh repeatedly throughout the lab session. Allie and Gemma notice the interaction and address the group of students by saying, "Guys, I don't think this is appropriate. Dr. Singh has been talking to you for a while and you're ignoring his instruction. This is very disrespectful of the professor, the cadavers, and the entire class to be honest. And it is Dr. Singh not Dr. Shing, by the way." One student responds to Allie and Gemma by saying, "Wow! Sorry! We just did not think it mattered that much. We will be quiet." After class, Allie and Gemma talk to Dr. Singh to discuss that incident and their plans to talk to the program director about the group's behavior.

Reflective pause

- What do you think of the interaction between the group of OT students and Dr. Singh?
- What do you feel about Allie and Gemma stepping up and supporting Dr. Singh?
- What would you perhaps have done differently?

Commentary on Case example 2.1

This scenario describes an unfortunate incident where a group of students violate class conduct by disrespecting the professor and the cadavers. The students are demonstrating unprofessional behaviors that may even violate the profession's code of ethics, such as the core value of dignity (i.e. valuing the worth of each person and showing behaviors of dignity) and the principle of fidelity (i.e. showing respect to clients). Allie and Gemma supporting the professor in this situation is not easy as they are, in a sense, correcting their peers. That said, it demonstrates an incredible allyship (and potentially even accompliceship) with the professor, who may not be as vocal as other professors in the program given his cultural background and personal traits. This case example also shows that allyship and accompliceship do not have to come from a trusted, known source. Any individual, group, or community can be an ally or accomplice.

Accompliceship

Accompliceship goes a step further than allyship. While allies offer support and solidarity, accomplices and individuals, communities, groups, and organizations take active risks in participating in dismantling systemic barriers of oppression (Jones, 2021). Accompliceship requires the element of risk-taking, challenging power structures, and using one's privilege to confront injustice and oppression directly, even if it challenges or disturbs the status of the accomplice(s) themselves. Beyond allyship, accompliceship involves more profound commitment and action in dismantling the structures that oppress an individual or group and often involves personal sacrifice and discomfort (Clemens, 2017).

Accomplices recognize that liberation is interconnected, and they arduously work alongside marginalized communities in their fight for freedom and justice. It's about being actively engaged; rather than simply standing on the sidelines as allies, accomplices are on the front lines in the fight for creating a more equitable society. The Coalition of Occupational Therapy Advocates for Diversity (COTAD) is an example of an organization that is an accomplice in the occupational therapy profession. COTAD actively pursues justice, equity, diversity, and inclusion work, avidly supporting various marginalized and underrepresented groups as issues arise. DiverseOT is another advocacy group calling for cultural responsiveness, social equity, and diversifying the OT profession by recruiting students from underrepresented communities.

CASE EXAMPLE 2.2: Cheyenne advocates, "Hair is not a dress code"

Dr. Taylor goes over the dress code while discussing lab instructions in the OT in Physical Dysfunction course. The dress code states that "hair must be kept neat and not appear unruly" but does not have any more specifics. Some students express concerns with the dress code but no one shares their concerns with Dr. Taylor. A few days later, Gemma starts wearing her hair differently, with no braids or twists; another girl undoes their dreadlocks, and another classmate straightens their curly hair. Cheyenne talks to the three students about the change in hairstyle. Gemma says, "Of course I am upset and I have issues with the policy but I don't want to 'rock the boat.' I just want to finish the course in peace." Cheyenne, in her role as the leader of the class's Student Organization for Occupational Therapy (SOTA), decides to talk to Dr. Taylor about the dress code. Dr. Taylor responds, "I understand completely, but I don't write the program policies. You can speak to the program director about that." Cheyenne meets with the program director and states, "Hair is not a dress code: it is a personal identity, a heritage, a racial pride." She then proposes establishing a student advisory board to weigh in on DEI+ issues related to the curriculum and program policies. The program director approves the suggestion and asks Cheyenne to discuss this with the class.

Reflective pause

- What is the problem here with the dress code?
- How do you view Cheyenne in this scenario?
- Have you faced a situation like this? If you have or not, what would you do in this situation?

Commentary on Case example 2.2

This scenario describes a common situation in that "unspoken rules" (things that are at times expected to be known, but someone unfamiliar with the situation might not be aware of) are barriers to individuals, groups, and communities that must be broken down with appropriate communication. In this scenario, the lack of details leaves a lot of gray areas, and unfortunately, we see some undesired effects. Students are code-switching to fit into the system and avoid trouble when truly they have no reason to be concerned. Or perhaps they do? It is critical for policies to be discussed thoroughly and spelled out to avoid miscommunication or unintended consequences.

Advocacy

Advocacy is the act of supporting or promoting a cause, idea, or policy. It involves speaking, writing, or acting in favor of something to influence public opinion or decision-making. Advocacy can take many forms, from grassroots activism to lobbying governments and organizations. Advocacy plays a crucial role in bringing about social, political, and environmental change by raising awareness, mobilizing communities, and pushing for policy reforms. Effective advocacy often requires strategic planning, collaboration, and persistence to achieve meaningful impact (Cullerton et al., 2018).

Below are some strategies students can use to enhance their sense of advocacy:

- Speak up and say something when you know it is not correct.
- Join your state OT association.
- Join your program advocacy groups (e.g. SOTA, COTAD).
- Participate in fundraising for advocacy causes (e.g. advocating for accessibility for students with limited mobility).

- Contact the university office for inclusion and diversity.
- Protest in a non-violent, peaceful way.
- Join and actively volunteer at a local non-profit community organization supporting a respective cause.
- Actively participate in state/national OT Hill Day.
- Contact local representatives and legislators.

CASE EXAMPLE 2.3: Amihan runs for AOTA student delegate
One day, in class, program director Dr. Cruz sets up an AOTA Boardroom to Classroom presentation—an event where the AOTA Board of Directors connects and converses with the students to foster student advocacy. During the presentation, a board member mentions the importance of students having a voice in the AOTA. After the presentation ends, Amihan, an aspiring student leader of East Asian descent, says that she will run for the Assembly of Student Delegates (ASD) as she believes the Asian and Pacific Islander community must have a voice in the association. Dr. Cruz tells Amihan that she is fully supportive and willing to assist her in her run for the ASD. Dr. Cruz tells Amihan, "I will happily provide you with any references needed. If you have any questions, please do not hesitate to ask." Amihan thanks her program director, Dr. Cruz, who was kindly supportive.

Reflective pause

- How do you think Dr. Cruz supporting Amihan in such a way makes her feel?
- How important is it to see representation in the occupational therapy profession, seeing practitioners and academicians who look like you, and why?
- Do you feel Dr. Cruz is an ally?

Commentary on Case example 2.3

This scenario describes the importance of representation and is an excellent example of an educator supporting a student. Amihan clearly states that she feels the Asian and Pacific Islander community must have a place in her national professional association. The scenario is also vital in that it shows the power of "planting the seed" in education. Dr. Cruz's utilizing the AOTA Boardroom to Classroom program to feature an AOTA board member virtually spurs Amihan to pursue her dreams and ambitions of running for the AOTA Assembly of Student Delegates.

Allyship, accompliceship, and advocacy on fieldwork

Individuals can also advocate for their own needs and rights; this is referred to as self-advocacy (American Psychological Association, 2018). While advocacy and self-advocacy are being discussed in the context of DEI+ they are important terms for students to know in general, particularly self-advocacy. The occupational therapy practitioner's role in promoting a client's self-advocacy, for example in support of individuals with disabilities, is a critical one that all OTs and OTAs must work on to ensure individuals are given the services they need. Allyship is an important strategy for promoting belonging and promotes social justice (Atwal *et al.*, 2021).

Fieldwork is a time to solidify the foundational principles learned within the OT didactic education. However, it is also a time of great uneasiness for students as the same transitional process that occurs when entering a program occurs with the Level I fieldwork educator. Self-advocacy is a critical tool during fieldwork, for students to optimize their learning.

> **CASE EXAMPLE 2.4: Malik reports racist remarks by the fieldwork educator**
>
> Malik is on the last day of his Level I experience in pediatrics. He overhears the fieldwork educator discussing a client with another co-worker. The fieldwork educator remarks that the child (client) is slow and does not know any better. "Her parents are just the wrong type of people—quite honestly, these people should not bring kids into the world. They are poor, uneducated, and can't afford children. They are just simply careless and don't care about their children."
>
> After overhearing this comment, Malik calls his academic fieldwork coordinator, Dr. Klein, and informs her of the details of this conversation. Malik states that he would not like to return to this site for his Level II fieldwork and capstone, "This stinks, Dr. Klein. I was enjoying my Level I experience until I heard those remarks. However, I no longer feel comfortable." Dr. Klein responds to Malik, "I understand how you feel and we will talk about this when you return to campus."

Reflective pause

- What in this scenario is wrong? Hint: there are multiple issues.
- What image of the parents came to mind? (Internally, reflect on this. Do you see it as a potential personal bias?)
- What should Malik do to handle this scenario professionally?

Commentary on Case example 2.4

This scenario is truly a situation you hate to see or hear of. Yet, unfortunately, it happens in the real world. The fieldwork educator in this scenario demonstrates many ethical violations and states racist stereotypes. The fieldwork educator also speaks about the child inappropriately, and the comments about the parents are unconscionable and should not be said. As a result of this situation, the student doesn't want to return to the placement. One problem has sullied an otherwise great overall experience and has had a catastrophic effect on the student. Also, the academic fieldwork coordinator will need to report this matter to the program director, Dr. Cruz, and determine a plan of action that may include terminating future placements at this facility.

Let's think about it

A few months into the MSOT program, Gemma has scheduled an advisement meeting with her advisor, Dr. Campbell, a Jamaican American faculty member who also teaches leadership development and advocacy. Gemma states, "I am doing great; my grades are excellent, and I am enjoying the program." Dr. Campbell responds, "That is wonderful to hear. Is there anything you would like to speak about today?" Gemma says, "Well, Dr. Campbell, as you know, I am greatly interested in accessibility. With that, I wanted to ask: why don't we have any students with disabilities? Additionally, our building is not that accessible." Dr. Campbell says, "I did not see that question coming today, but it's a great question. Gemma, I can tell you that we do have individuals with unseen disabilities in our program, but I cannot disclose those details as it is not my place. I'm sure you understand. Regarding the building, as an OT faculty, we have made some recommendations to Dean Thompson and she expressed that the university is addressing some things. At the same time, I do see your point on students with disabilities, and I will bring this up with the program director Dr. Cruz."

Reflective thinking

- What do you think about this interaction and Gemma advocating for students with disabilities?

Critical thinking questions

- Why are allyship and mentorship essential in occupational therapy academic and clinical environments?
- How can we work together as students and faculty staff to ensure an inclusive classroom environment?
- Explore strategies to foster allyship and mentorship.

Action-oriented thinking

- Think of one action Gemma can take to address her interest in accessibility.
- Think of one further action Gemma can take on a programmatic or campus level to further advocate for students with disabilities.

HOT TAKE

Allyship is risky. It is safer not to engage. After all, I can't fix the world.

Read: "Allyship, antiracism and the strength of weak ties: A barber, a professor and an entrepreneur walk into a room" (Terry, 2021).

References

American Association of Colleges of Nursing. (2024). Allyship. www.aacnnursing.org/5b-tool-kit/themes/allyship

American Occupational Therapy Association. (2024). Multicultural, Diversity, and Inclusion Network. www.aota.org/community/volunteer-groups

American Psychological Association. (2018). APA Dictionary of Psychology. https://dictionary.apa.org/self-advocacy

Arif, S., Afolabi, T., Mitrzyk, B. M., Thomas, T. F., et al. (2022). Engaging in authentic allyship as part of our professional development. American Journal of Pharmaceutical Education, 86(5), 8690. https://doi.org/10.5688/ajpe8690

Atwal, A., Sriram, V., & McKay, E. A. (2021). Making a difference: Belonging, diversity, and inclusion in occupational therapy. *British Journal of Occupational Therapy, 84*(11), 671–672. https://doi.org/10.1177/03080226211031797

Burgess, A., van Diggele, C., Roberts, C., & Mellis, C. (2020). Feedback in the clinical setting. *BMC Medical Education, 20*(S2). https://doi.org/10.1186/s12909-020-02280-5

Clemens, C. (2017). Ally or accomplice? The language of activism. Learning for Justice. www.learningforjustice.org/magazine/ally-or-accomplice-the-language-of-activism

Cullen, J. P., Ellinas, E., & Lautenberger, D. (2022). *A Guide to Allyship.* Association of American Medical Colleges. www.aamc.org/media/52121/download

Cullerton, K., Donnet, T., Lee, A., & Gallegos, D. (2018). Effective advocacy strategies for influencing government nutrition policy: A conceptual model. *International Journal of Behavioral Nutrition and Physical Activity, 15*(1), 83. https://doi.org/10.1186/s12966-018-0716-y

De Souza, L. & Schmader, T. (2025). When people do allyship: A typology of allyship action. *Personality and Social Psychology Review, 29*(1), 3–31. doi: 10.1177/10888683241232732

Jones, J. C. (2021). We need accomplices, not allies in the fight for an equitable geoscience. *AGU Advances, 2,* e2021AV000482. https://doi.org/10.1029/2021AV000482

Nilsson, I. & Townsend, E. (2010). Occupational justice–bridging theory and practice. *Scandinavian Journal of Occupational Therapy, 17*(1), 57–63. https://doi.org/10.3109/11038120903287182

Terry, P. E. (2021). Allyship, antiracism and the strength of weak ties: A barber, a professor and an entrepreneur walk into a room. *American Journal of Health Promotion, 35*(2), 163–167. https://doi.org/10.1177/0890117120982201

CHAPTER 3

Bias and Microaggressions

"Professional means proper English"

Razan Hamed PhD., OTR/L

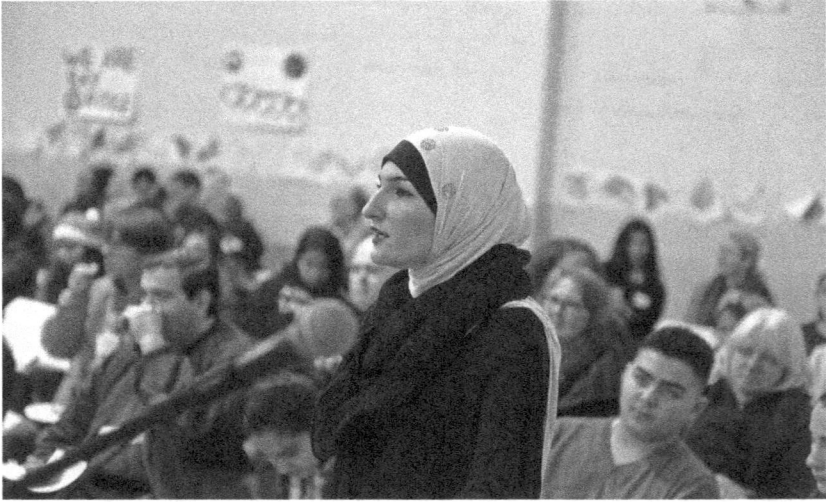

Chapter overview

This chapter introduces bias and its related constructs, such as micro-aggression, discrimination, and oppression, and their influence on one's professional identity. Examples of interactions involving both active and passive forms of microaggressions and implicit/explicit bias are explored through a case-based lens. The chapter discusses strategies to navigate daily interactions and opportunities to recognize bias and privilege and build skills for advocacy, allyship, and accompliceship. Students are invited to reflect on their own biases and how harmful they can be to others in daily and professional interactions.

Content

- All things bias, Case example 3.1: Microaggressions.
- Bias and difficult conversations in the classroom, Case example 3.2: "Use proper English, Gemma!"
- Bias and intersectionality, Case example 3.3: "It is against my beliefs to work with the LGBTQIA+ community."
- Let's think about it.

Objectives

1. Identify concepts related to bias and microaggression within academic and clinical education.
2. Describe behaviors that are associated with bias and microaggression.
3. Apply strategies to address bias, difficult conversations, and discriminatory learning environments.
4. Recognize the connection between bias and empathy.
5. Recognize the role of intersectionality in understanding and projecting bias.

Storyline snapshot

The students are diving into their journey at occupational therapy school. They are taking courses together, working on group assignments, meeting with academic advisors, and attending various professional activities. Classroom conversations are a mix of new knowledge, personal and professional growth, and insight into issues within the world of DEI+. Other conversations are happening over meals, extracurricular activities while commuting, and at other campus corners. Regardless of where these conversations are happening, they are bringing another kind of growth—growth of the mind and self. Students are reflecting on their views of themselves, people, communities, and the world. These insights are not always pleasant but they are the steps that pave the way for bias-free spaces where everyone feels they belong.

In this chapter, Allie and Gemma work on a key class presentation on leadership—same presentation, same grade, different feedback.

Characters in this chapter (see character matrix in Appendix 2 for details)

- Allie
- Gemma
- Dr. Boyle
- Dr. Moore
- Yara
- Elizabeth
- Cheyenne
- Dr. Gallagher
- Hana

Introduction

Change will not come if we wait for some other person or some other time. We are the ones we've been waiting for. We are the change that we seek.

BARACK OBAMA, FORMER US PRESIDENT

Bias is part of being human. We all have biases, and there are no exceptions. However, when we take on the role of a healthcare professional we are held accountable for not projecting these biases toward others. Unfortunately, healthcare practitioners, including those in occupational therapy, exhibit similar levels of implicit biases as the general population, leading to inconsistent client care (FitzGerald & Hurst, 2017). Research shows that occupational therapy students can be biased toward people who are overweight (Friedman & VanPuymbrouck, 2019), older (Friedman & VanPuymbrouck, 2021a; Giles *et al.*, 2002), or disabled (Friedman & VanPuymbrouck, 2021b). Inspecting our biases is critical for professional communication and delivering ethical client-centered care. Bias is an automatic irrational belief about an individual or a group of people who possess certain traits or characteristics. All students must recognize their biases and contemplate how they shape daily interactions with others within personal and professional environments. It is important to recognize the impact our interactions impose on other people's lives when our biases are not checked or curtailed. Most people do not recognize their bias and may deeply believe that they act in good faith and with sincere intentions. Normalizing biases can result in empathy decline toward others and can perpetuate the traumas and marginalization of diverse communities (e.g. racial, disabled, LGBTQIA+).

All things bias

Microaggressions are various actions related to bias and are defined as indirect and subtle insults in daily conversations from people who are associated with power toward people from marginalized groups (Sue *et al.*, 2009). Microaggressions are projections of personal biases, assumptions, and prejudice toward individuals, groups, or communities. Forms of microaggressions include microinvalidation (i.e. negating someone's experiences), microassaults (i.e. intentional attacks), or microinsults (i.e. insensitive remarks or gestures; Sue *et al.*, 2007). Microaggressive behaviors towards students include dismissive looks, denigrating comments, demeaning gestures, and disrespectful jokes or snubs. Albeit subtle, microaggressions are harmful and can damage targeted students' well-being and professional identity. Studies show that microaggression can perpetuate stereotypes, undermine mental and physical health outcomes, and reduce work productivity (Anderson *et al.*, 2022; Sue *et al.*, 2008). Occupational therapy students experiencing microaggressions in didactic or clinical education may feel slighted, isolated, or excluded, which can affect their ability to study, communicate, and focus on class interactions (Burks & Olson, 2023; Solorzano *et al.*, 2000).

Fortunately, identifying and articulating our biases is a trainable ability that starts by recognizing our biases about others by paying attention to our thoughts about a particular group (e.g. recognizing that you "secretly" believe that Black students are not as hard-working as non-Black students). Understanding how our behaviors (no matter how well intended) can hurt others in daily interactions is an essential next step to reducing bias. Reflecting and verbalizing how our behavior has affected someone else can be validating to that person's experience. Hence, it is important not to trivialize the effect of our "well-intended" behavior on someone's feelings.

Table 3.1: Terms related to bias and microaggressions

Term	Description	Example
Implicit bias	Unconscious beliefs that stem from associating a group of people with a particular trait. The person inadvertently projects stereotypes, generalizations, or insults without overtly using offensive language. Implicit bias perpetuates overt bias and affects people's mental health.	An instructor assumes that Black students in the classroom would be interested in tutoring support offered by the OT program.
Explicit bias	Irrational assumptions or misconceptions about someone's abilities or worth. These are damaging to people's self-worth and health.	Consistently rejecting Hispanic applicants from an OT program due to anticipating their inability to succeed.
Micro-aggressions	Subtle verbal or non-verbal insults in daily interactions directed at individuals of marginalized communities. Can be damaging to students' self-esteem and well-being.	Complimenting an Asian student for speaking English with no accent.
Micro-invalidation	Language or behaviors that negate, minimize, or dismiss someone's experiences, thoughts, sentiments, or feelings. Microinvalidation can undermine trust in learning spaces and limit effective communication between students and educators.	Telling someone that they are overthinking or overreacting to a comment directed toward them.
Micro-assaults	Conscious and intended actions or attacks meant to deliberately but subtly offend, target, or hurt someone.	Addressing someone's comment while looking at someone else or looking away, or rolling eyes while someone is talking.
Micro-insults	Demeaning comments or language used to convey the idea that someone is inferior or subpar because of their culture or heritage.	Telling a student of color that they were very lucky to be accepted into a competitive program.
Stereotypes	Unchecked automatic beliefs about a group or community.	The belief that people who are overweight are less intelligent.

Note: The terms defined in this table are common at the time of writing this chapter. New terms may emerge to reflect new realities and sociopolitical contexts.

CASE EXAMPLE 3.1: Microaggressions

The students are completing a group assignment in Dr. Moore's class, Introduction to Occupational Therapy. Yara, self-identified as a second-generation Moroccan-American Muslim, is working with four other students on a presentation for the first time in the semester. The students do not know each other very well. The assignment requires the students to use the occupational therapy practice framework to highlight the role of religion and spirituality in coping with disability. The students in the group share how their faith practices perceive illness and disability. Yara shares that Islam calls for people to care for themselves, seek treatment when they fall sick, and to attend to their families and daily occupations. She also shares that Islam condemns blaming God or the deity for disabilities and calls for resilience and patience. When Yara is done, Elizabeth, a self-identified Catholic, comments, "Wow! Interesting, I always thought Islam was more of a surrender-to-your-fate kind of ideology." Yara answers, "Hmmm, well, it is not an ideology: Islam is a major religion, and it calls people to have faith in God and fate, not surrender when sick." Cheyenne, self-identified as Indigenous, responds, "Thank you for sharing this, Yara; I appreciate it. I also think your accent is beautiful. When did you first come to the US?" Yara responds, "I did not know I have an accent but thank you! I was born and raised in Allentown, Pennsylvania, but I am bilingual, so you may be picking up my other tongue."

Reflective pause

- Are the comments made by Elizabeth or Cheyenne offensive?
- What is the difference between ideology and religion?
- What do you think of Yara's responses to her classmates?
- Reflect on the first time you worked with your classmates on a group assignment. What was the group dynamic like? Were any of the conversations you had with your group mates challenging or uncomfortable?

Commentary on Case example 3.1

The scenario describes a common situation in the early stages of occupational therapy studies, where students work together on group assignments. When students are not familiar with each other, conversations may feel engaging and warm, or they may feel awkward and stiff. The scenario here reflects a common stereotype-affirming conversation about Muslims who commonly face microaggressions in occupational therapy education and practice (Khan, 2023). The phrases "this is interesting" and "creed" are based on preconceptions or inaccurate information about Islam. Although Elizabeth is careful not to offend Yara, and Yara's response does not show that she is offended, one cannot rule out that she was not comfortable with the question. An alternative way of asking the same question would have been, "Wow! That is interesting to me because I am not familiar with your faith. I am curious, but I do not want to offend you. Do you mind if I asked more questions about this?" Similarly, Cheyenne's comment about Yara's accent is probably meant as a compliment, which is not the problem. It is the assumption behind the question that may offend the other person. It is usually safe to preface your question with your positionality (i.e. the factors, background, or personal traits that shaped your opinion or led you to ask a certain question).

Bias and difficult conversations in the classroom

Bias and microaggressions may lead to difficult conversations in the class-room and challenging interactions with the instructor and classmates (Eisen, 2020). If poorly facilitated, these conversations can be damaging to class rapport, learning, and a sense of student community. For example, when lecture content contains bias-tainted or stereotype-affirming case studies (e.g. a Hispanic single mother with less than a high school education), it may create a hostile learning environment by potentially offending some students. Although creating an inclusive learning space is mainly the instructor's responsibility, students can have an active role in addressing incidents of bias and microaggressions. Students may not feel comfortable approaching these conversations, fearing peer judgment, retaliation by the instructor, or rupturing classroom cohesiveness. However, when students do address these conversations, it promotes mindful classroom conversations, empowers other students with similar concerns, and creates opportunities for peer growth.

To navigate difficult conversations, students can follow the steps below:

1. Remind yourself that you have the right to express your thoughts and opinions.
2. Select a time when you feel comfortable sharing your input (e.g. in-class versus privately with the instructor).

3. Respectfully address the instructor and ask to share a perspective that is meant to foster mindful and inclusive classroom discussions (e.g. "May I share a perspective on the case study presented?").

4. Clearly describe the problematic class content or comments made by other students rather than the person themselves (e.g. the case study presented in class rather than the presenter). Share factors, evidence, or research to back up your point, and provide context.

5. Clearly and concisely describe the reasons you find the content problematic (e.g. over-generalization or stereotype-perpetuating phrases).

6. Clearly articulate your thoughts and feelings (e.g. "I was disappointed with the example given on this population/culture/ethnic group because it was over-generalizing and stereotypical").

7. Describe your positionality (i.e. personal reasons, background, or unique experiences that shaped your opinion: "As a Hispanic-identifying student, I feel the case study was offensive to my ethnic group").

8. If you can, articulate alternative language or content for future instances.

9. Remember that the point of sharing is to foster a mindful co-learning space with others, not to shame or blame your instructor or classmates

CASE EXAMPLE 3.2: "Use proper English, Gemma!"

Gemma and Allie worked together on a presentation for Dr. Boyle's class on leadership and management. Dr. Boyle then meets with the students to share feedback on presentation delivery and commends Allie and Gemma for a clear and smooth presentation. She then makes a few suggestions for improvement, including using proper English and professional language. She explains that "Using professional language is an important communication skill in clinical practice, so next time, try to sound more professional and less casual." Both Gemma and Allie are confused and ask a follow-up question about that. Dr. Boyle responds while looking at Gemma, "Well, I noticed that you were slightly informal while presenting and used casual English. We present ourselves as professionals who are expected to communicate clearly with proper English and correct grammar. I am sorry if I sound harsh but it is my job to give you feedback on your professional behaviors so you can succeed in the real world." Both students nod politely, thank the instructor, and return to class. While in the hallway, Allie, still confused, asks Gemma what she thinks about the interaction with Dr. Boyle. Gemma responds, "I think she does not like my English." Allie responds, "That did not feel right. You should have said something, Gemma."

Reflective pause

- What do you think Dr. Boyle means by "casual English", and why does she address Gemma with that?
- Do you think Gemma should say something to Dr. Boyle? Why or why not?
- What suggestions would you make for Gemma to address this incident?
- Do you think Allie could/should say something to Dr. Boyle?

Commentary on Case example 3.2

This scenario describes an incident where comments made by the instructor are offensive to a student. The comments are microaggressive because they target Gemma and insinuate that she does not speak proper English, probably given her racial identity. Although Dr. Boyle is sharing professional advice on the student's performance and linking it to effective communication in clinical practice, she may cause emotional or professional harm to the student. As a self-identified person of color, Gemma uses African American Vernacular English (AAVE), a form of English widely used by Black Americans and Black Canadians. AAVE is not colloquial, casual, or standard English with poor grammar but rather a distinct version of English spoken proudly by many members of the Black and African American community (Pullum, 1999). Gemma may have not felt comfortable or confident at the time to discuss Dr. Boyle's remark, but a conversation is necessary to address this incident. Although not directly affected, Allie felt that the comments made by Dr. Boyle were not appropriate and Gemma seemed to be upset by them. Recognizing and identifying harm done to classmates of color is one step toward allyship and advocacy (see Chapter 2).

Bias and intersectionality

Many students may have a basic understanding of issues related to race, ethnicity, culture, disability, and other DEI+ constructs. Education is meant not only to prepare students for a professional career but also to transform them into autonomous, reflective, lifelong learners who solve problems (Mezirow, 1997). While interacting with students of diverse backgrounds, occupational therapy school is a good time to gain insight and awareness on these issues in preparation for their future role as clinicians (see Chapter 8). Identifying one's biases can enhance empathy and future professional skills in clinical practice. Building bias-free communication skills is necessary in interprofessional collaboration, working with clients and their caregivers, and working with colleagues and staff.

Our biases can shape our views of the world and, consequently, our behaviors toward others. These behaviors may directly or indirectly cause harm to someone's mental and physical health (FitzGerald & Hurst, 2017). As future occupational therapy practitioners, students must check their biases and reflect on how their preconceived knowledge contributes to their biases. Students must also acknowledge other components associated with bias, such as privilege and power. For example, students may not recognize an incident of bias when it occurs because they have not had similar experiences in the past due to their privilege (i.e. favorable status) related to race, gender, skin tone, ability status, weight, faith, height, socioeconomic status, family status, family heritage, and other personal factors shaping their view of the world.

Bias and intersectionality in the classroom

Students must also recognize their intersectionality and how it shapes their biases or their ability to minimize them (Hill Collins, 1993). Intersectionality is defined as the interplay between various personal factors and how they shape experiences of power, privilege, and oppression in someone's life (Crenshaw, 2019). For example, if a student identifies with a minoritized, marginalized, or underrepresented group that historically or presently faces prejudice, discrimination, or bigotry then they are more likely to subconsciously recognize bias and incidents of discrimination (Williams *et al.*, 2021). And if a student identifies with a majority group or a historically and presently privileged group, then they are less likely to subconsciously recognize bias and microaggressions. This does not mean that the students with power and privilege are not themselves sometimes vilified or do not have good intentions; it just means that they are less likely to relate to an experience that is not (or is less) associated with their status or heritage (Clark & Spanierman, 2018)

Additionally, recognizing our intersectionality helps identify environmental factors that are hindering or facilitating our growth and success. Students must reflect on others' intersectionality and the various layers of diversity that shape their behaviors and health outcomes (Hamed, 2020). Our implicit biases stem from our current and past experiences, which are greatly shaped by our intersectionality. Therefore, reflecting on our intersectionality can be essential to recognizing our own biases when interacting with others. It can also help recognize incidents of bias when witnessing others being discriminated against. Ultimately, this insight and awareness will prepare students to handle incidents of bias and micro-aggression, taking an ally or accomplice role, or advocating for inclusive learning and working spaces.

The Macro-Micro Model of Diversity (MMMD)

One should consider the intersectionality at the macro and micro levels of their diverse experience. The Macro-Micro Level of Diversity (Hamed, 2020) describes the various levels of our diverse existence and how they influence our daily occupations and interactions with others in our environments. It also describes how the interplay of these layers and other surrounding factors within our communities shape our success and daily function. The model describes four levels: the macro layers (community and culture) and micro layers (individual and core) of our diverse backgrounds and experiences as defined in the occupational therapy practice framework (American Occupational Therapy Association, 2020a).

At the macro level, our diversity factors are more recognizable and distinct from others. For example, the *community* layer recognizes groups of people with similar traits, history, or status (e.g. race, ethnicity, socio-economic status, immigration status, ability, language, etc.) and is affected by external environments and contexts (e.g. social policies, legislations, economy). Therefore, our traits at this level (e.g. race) are greatly affected by social and governmental policies (e.g. access to healthcare). The other macro layer is *culture*, which recognizes shared cultural beliefs and values among a group of people (e.g. family traditions) and is greatly affected by *social systems* (e.g. gender norms), which eventually shape our community participation.

At the micro levels, our diversity is less recognizable at face value and highly unique to individual experiences. For example, the *individual layer* recognizes our occupations, body traits, habits, and roles. Our individuality is greatly influenced by *life events* that ultimately shape how we navigate our daily activities and functional goals. Finally, the *core layer* recognizes the most subtle level of our diverse existence as unique functional beings, such as our gender identity, self-expression, and personal values, and is greatly affected by the passage of time and temporal factors. This most personal layer of diversity molds our well-being, life meaning, and quality of life.

The different layers of diversity mold our intersectionality which in turn influences our biases, sense of empathy, ability to recognize bias, and aptitude for allyship and advocacy. Collectively this interaction shapes professional communication skills in clinical practice. Consider the *intersectionality map* below to reflect on your intersectionality as described by the MMMD.

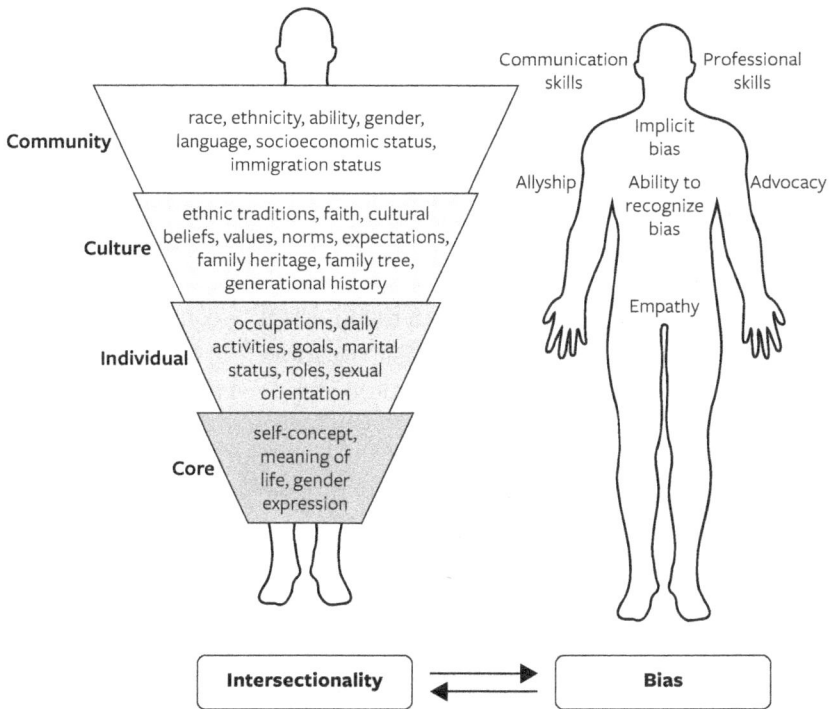

Figure 3.1: Intersectionality and bias (adapted from Hamed, 2020)

CASE EXAMPLE 3.3: "It is against my beliefs to work with the LGBTQIA+ community"

Students are starting their first simulated fieldwork experience in physical dysfunctions. Dr. Gallagher, the fieldwork coordinator who also teaches kinesiology, is showing the students a video of a case study. The video shows the client being treated for a shoulder injury by the occupational therapy assistant at the client's home. She describes the client in the case study as a 36-year-old male high-school music teacher who lives in an urban area with his husband and two dogs. The students break into pairs to work on identifying occupation-based activities for the treatment plan. Hana overhears another student saying to her classmate, "I don't know, I wouldn't treat a gay man. I can't, it's against my religious beliefs to work with anyone from the LGBTQIA+ community." Hana turns around and says to the student, "I don't think we have an option if we are treating people. Our code of ethics says that we need to treat everyone fairly, doesn't it?" The other student responds, "I would just decline to treat the client, it's my right." Hana feels uncomfortable with the response and shares that her cousin identifies as gay and she can't imagine someone declining to treat him because of his sexual orientation. She talks to Dr. Gallagher after class about this interaction.

Reflective pause

- What do you think of Hana's response to the student's comments on not treating someone from the LGBTQIA+ community?
- How would you react in a similar situation?
- Do you think Dr. Gallagher should step into this conversation? Why or why not?

Commentary on Case example 3.3

This scenario describes a conversation that contains a personal bias against members of the LGBTQIA+ community. Although the comments by the student are harmful, the awareness of personal biases and boundaries is important when treating clients. While our code of ethics calls for justice in our practice (i.e. treating all clients fairly and equitably) the principle of nonmaleficence (i.e. avoiding harm) urges practitioners to refrain from actions that cause harm or wrongdoing to clients (American

Occupational Therapy Association, 2020b). In this case, a practitioner's personal biases may consciously or subconsciously result in ineffective or careless practice. Although Hana feels comfortable challenging the comments in class, not all students have the same feeling about addressing conversations like this one. That said, if students do not want to confront the commenter or address the comments directly, some may opt for asking tone-neutral questions (e.g. with no judgment) that may help provide clarification or start a reflective conversation. If made aware, Dr. Gallagher can address the issues of bias in light of the AOTA code of ethics' principles and values.

Let's think about it

Reflect on Figure 3.1 earlier and the Macro-Micro Model of Diversity. Then complete the intersectionality wheel below (Figure 3.2) to reflect on how your layers of diversity shape your identity and your interactions with other people in your world. In your reflection, consider how you perceive your diversity components by using the scale below. After scoring each component, add the total score for each section (e.g. community, core).

1 = Least favorable status
2 = Somewhat unfavorable status
3 = Neutral or not sure
4 = Somewhat favorable status
5 = Most favorable status

Recap

The intersectionality wheel describes various components of human diversity categorized based on the Macro-Micro Model of Diversity (Hamed, 2020). Our intersectionalities can shape how we see and feel about others in external contexts (e.g. community and culture) and how we see and feel about ourselves intrinsically (e.g. individual and core). These perceptions may influence our interactions with others in personal and professional communication. Our intersectionality may make us relate to others' experiences at a higher or lesser level and hence increase or decrease our sense of empathy toward their experiences. For example, if you identify as a Black woman with a disability, you are subconsciously more likely to understand and empathize with the experiences of other Black women with disabilities.

The intricacies of being a member of a historically persecuted and oppressed racial group (i.e. Black), experiencing gender-specific biases (i.e. women), and facing barriers to access and equity (i.e. disability) can be more relatable to others with the same intersectionality (i.e. Black women with disabilities). This does not mean that people from other racial groups, gender identities, or ability statuses do not relate or empathize with Black women with disability. It simply means that the more similar the intersectionality is, the more likely we are to be more empathic and less biased. If we bring this connection to our consciousness then we can deter our biases toward others with different intersectionalities. This is very important in your role as a future clinician when interacting with clients and families with different intersectionalities. In this exercise, you can reflect on the interplay between your intersectionality and your implicit biases.

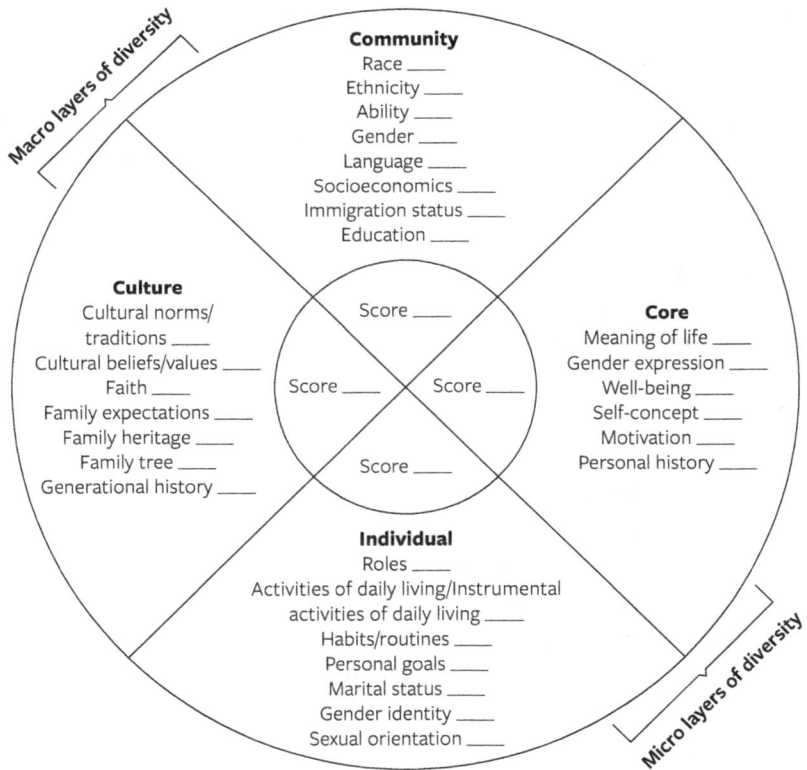

Figure 3.2: Intersectionality wheel

Reflective thinking

- How do you feel about your intersectionality after completing the intersectionality wheel in Figure 3.2?
- Describe how your intersectionality shapes your biases.

Critical thinking

- If you were able to change one aspect of your intersectionality, what would that be and why? How will that influence your views of others and the world?

Action-oriented thinking

- Find a classmate who is open to sharing their intersectionality wheel. Compare yours to theirs and find common and different components of your intersectionalities.

HOT TAKE

Discuss how microaggressions can perpetuate systemic racism, White supremacy, and inequities in healthcare.

Suggested reading to navigate this question: "How microaggressions reinforce and perpetuate systemic racism in the United States" (Skinner-Dorkenoo *et al.*, 2021).

References

American Occupational Therapy Association. (2020a). Occupational Therapy Code of Ethics. *American Journal of Occupational Therapy, 74*(3), 7413410005p1–7413410005p13. https://doi.org/10.5014/ajot.2020.74S3006

American Occupational Therapy Association. (2020b). Occupational therapy practice framework: Domain and process. *American Journal of Occupational Therapy, 74*(2), 7412410010p1–7412410010p87. https://doi.org/10.5014/ajot.2020.74S2001

Anderson, N., Lett, E., Asabor, E. N., Hernandez, A. L., *et al.* (2022). The association of microaggressions with depressive symptoms and institutional satisfaction among a national cohort of medical students. *Journal of General Internal Medicine, 37*(2), 298–307. https://doi.org/10.1007/s11606-021-06786-6

Burks, K. A. & Olson, L. (2023). Let's talk about it: Addressing microaggressions in occupational therapy education. *American Journal of Occupational Therapy*, 77(3), 7703347010. https://doi.org/10.5014/ajot.2023.050125

Clark, D. A. & Spanierman, L. (2018). "'I Didn't Know That Was Racist': Costs of Racial Micro-aggressions to White People." In G. C. Torino, D. P. Rivera, C. M. Capodilupo, K. L. Nadal, & D. W. Sue (eds), *Microaggression Theory* (first edition, pp.138–155). Wiley. https://doi.org/10.1002/9781119466642.ch9

Crenshaw, K. (2019). *On Intersectionality: Essential Writings*. New Press.

Eisen, D. B. (2020). Combating the "too sensitive" argument: A demonstration that captures the complexity of microaggressions. *Teaching Sociology*, 48(3), 231–243. https://doi.org/10.1177/0092055X20930338

FitzGerald, C. & Hurst, S. (2017). Implicit bias in healthcare professionals: A systematic review. *BMC Medical Ethics*, 18(1), 19. https://doi.org/10.1186/s12910-017-0179-8

Friedman, C. & VanPuymbrouck, L. H. (2019). Anti-fat bias of occupational therapy students. *Journal of Occupational Therapy Education*, 3(4). https://doi.org/10.26681/jote.2019.030406

Friedman, C. & VanPuymbrouck, L. (2021a). Ageism and ableism: Unrecognized biases in occupational therapy students. *Physical & Occupational Therapy in Geriatrics*, 39(4), 354–369. https://doi.org/10.1080/02703181.2021.1880531

Friedman, C. & VanPuymbrouck, L. (2021b). Impact of occupational therapy education on students' disability attitudes: A longitudinal study. *American Journal of Occupational Therapy*, 75(4), 7504180090. https://doi.org/10.5014/ajot.2021.047423

Giles, L. C., Paterson, J. E., Butler, S. J., & Stewart, J. J. (2002). Ageism among health professionals: A Comparison of clinical educators and students in physical and occupational therapy. *Physical & Occupational Therapy in Geriatrics*, 21(2), 15–26. https://doi.org/10.1080/J148v21n02_02

Hamed, R. (2020). "Addressing Diversity in Occupational Therapy Assessment." In P. Kramer & N. Grampurohit (eds), *Hinojosa and Kramer's Evaluation in Occupational Therapy: Obtaining and Interpreting Data* (fifth edition, pp.157–166). AOTA Press.

Hill Collins, P. (1993). Toward a new vision: Race, class, and gender as categories of analysis and connection. *Race, Sex & Class*, 1(1), 25–45.

Khan, S. (2023). The impact of microaggressions on occupational performance for Muslims. *British Journal of Occupational Therapy*, 86 (12), 791–793. https://doi.org/10.1177/03080226231188010

Mezirow, J. (1997). Transformative learning: Theory to practice. *New Directions for Adult and Continuing Education*, 1997(74), 5–12. https://doi.org/10.1002/ace.7401

Pullum, G. (1999). "African American Vernacular English is not Standard English with Mistakes." In R. S. Wheeler, *The Workings of Language: From Prescriptions to Perspectives* (pp.39–58). Praeger.

Skinner-Dorkenoo, A. L., Sarmal, A., André, C. J., & Rogbeer, K. G. (2021). How microaggressions reinforce and perpetuate systemic racism in the United States. *Perspectives on Psychological Science*, 16(5), 903–925. https://doi.org/10.1177/17456916211002543

Solorzano, D., Ceja, M., & Yosso, T. (2000). Critical race theory, racial microaggressions, and campus racial climate: The experiences of African American college students. *Journal of Negro Education*, 69(1/2), 60–73.

Sue, D. W., Capodilupo, C. M., Torino, G. C., Bucceri, J. M., *et al.* (2007). Racial microaggressions in everyday life: Implications for clinical practice. *American Psychologist*, 62(4), 271–286. https://doi.org/10.1037/0003-066X.62.4.271

Sue, D. W., Capodilupo, C. M., & Holder, A. M. B. (2008). Racial microaggressions in the life experience of Black Americans. *Professional Psychology: Research and Practice*, 39(3), 329–336. https://doi.org/10.1037/0735-7028.39.3.329

Sue, D. W., Lin, A. I., Torino, G. C., Capodilupo, C. M., & Rivera, D. P. (2009). Racial microaggressions and difficult dialogues on race in the classroom. *Cultural Diversity and Ethnic Minority Psychology*, 15(2), 183–190. https://doi.org/10.1037/a0014191

Williams, M. T., Ching, T. H. W., & Gallo, J. (2021). Understanding aggression and microaggressions by and against people of colour. *Cognitive Behaviour Therapist*, 14, e25. https://doi.org/10.1017/S1754470X21000234

CHAPTER 4

Privilege and Critical Consciousness

"Don't worry about it, I'll buy"

Vikram Pagpatan EdD., OTR/L, FAOTA

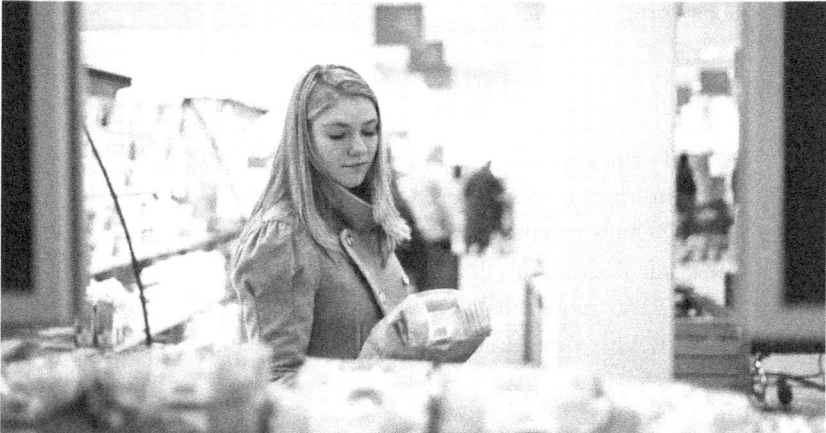

Chapter overview

Privilege can be a societal or inherent token that can drastically impact all facets of the healthcare process and so it is an important variable to consider for the occupational therapy student in education, advocacy, research, and practice. The awareness of privilege requires cognizant analysis, beyond what can be seen or measured. In this chapter, we introduce privilege as a multifaceted construct, with a focus on culture, race, access, socioeconomics, health literacy, and gender, which can be correlational to instances of bias and inequities within healthcare. Additionally, we provide opportunities for reflection and introspection as we discuss how the direct and indirect presence of privilege can influence social communication skills, sense of community and belonging, ethical and moral conflicts, professionalism and e-professionalism, and the developing clinical reasoning skills of the occupational therapy student and practitioner as they relate to community and client interactions.

Content

- Recognizing privilege as a social determinant of health.
- Critical consciousness, Case example 4.1: Malik and Christopher—"I feel as if we can relate, you know?"
- Recognizing factors related to privilege, Case example 4.2: Jamie talks to Dr. Campbell—"I don't understand what happened with Malik earlier this week."
- Let's think about it.

Objectives

1. Identify the aspects of privilege and power and how they affect daily interactions for an OTA/OT student.
2. Describe how privilege affects professional communication within the clinical and non-clinical space.
3. Apply strategies to utilize/leverage/address privilege in the classroom, fieldwork interactions, and capstone experiences.

Storyline snapshot

Jamie is walking into class after getting out of the subway and notices Malik at the corner. Jamie asks if Malik wants to grab some coffee and breakfast before heading into their morning neuroscience class and knows of a local coffee shop nearby where they could go. Malik kindly refuses by stating, "Thanks Jamie, I already had something to eat at home, but I'll walk with you" to which Jamie insists and replies with, "Don't worry about it, I'll buy it!" This interaction does not sit well with Malik and he walks away, headed towards school. Jamie and Malik get along very well in class and share many similar post-graduate aspirations. Jamie feels confused from what happened that morning and looks for an opportunity to talk to Malik throughout the day. Later that afternoon, they both sit in a guest presentation for travel occupational therapy services from a national recruiter during a break within a lab course. Although Malik feels highly inspired by the opportunities of the experience, he continues to be fixated on staying within his community as he knows that's where he would make the most impact and would feel safe doing so. During a group break in their lab class, Malik expresses his thoughts on travel therapy to his lab partner, Christopher. Jamie overhears and doesn't understand why Malik wouldn't want an opportunity to explore different places and even makes what she believes to be a humorous comment to Malik stating, "Is it because you're Black!?"

Characters in this chapter (see character matrix in Appendix 2 for details)

- Malik
- Jamie
- Christopher
- Dr. Campbell

Introduction

The more privilege you have, the more opportunity you have. The more opportunity you have, the more responsibility you have.

NOAM CHOMSKY

The World Health Organization defines social determinants of health (SDOH) as non-medical factors, forces, systems, and/or conditions under which people are born, grow, work, and live that shape conditions of daily life that influence health outcomes (World Health Organization, 2025). SDOH greatly impact how occupations are formed, judged, and inextricably connected throughout a person's life (Hacker *et al.* 2022). They encompass a broad range of social, economic, and environmental factors that influence an individual's occupations, health outcomes, and quality of life, in potentially harmful or beneficial ways. They are not experienced or accessed equally by individuals and can be adopted as generational, cultural, societal, and communal customs that are not always inclusive, equitable, or diverse regarding options and choices. For example, a single parent raising a child with lower socioeconomic status may not prioritize higher education as a future goal for their child's education, as immediate pressures of food, shelter, and employment may be held in higher regard based on the perception of privilege, survivability, and social class. These determinants are highly interconnected and correlated to the impact they have on any given individual's health, wellness, and occupation. In other words, where we work, live, and rest, and our access to resources and services, have a direct correlation to the viability of our health and wellness (Windsor *et al.*, 2022).

In both negative and positive ways, SDOH shape individual experiences, roles, rituals, routines, and behaviors and are highly influential in how health-related decisions are made. These non-medical factors can impact everyday life and are often not based on volitional control as they can encompass conditions in which individuals are born, and influence how they are raised, what they are exposed to, and what resources they have access to. For example, access to education, social support systems, employment opportunities, a sense of safety, and physically and emotionally nurturing/supportive contexts can all be considered SDOH that also directly shape occupational performance throughout an array of life stages. This chapter delves into an often overlooked social determinant of health—privilege—and why, when, and how occupational therapy students can use their understanding of privilege as a form of clinical and critical reasoning within education, research, and practice (Doll *et al.*, 2023).

Thus, the occupational therapy student must be cognizant of how integrating critical consciousness as a component of clinical and critical reasoning skills can be utilized not only to reflect on their awareness of their SDOH and factors of privilege/non-privilege but also to support their clients in their willingness to recognize and combat their health inequities and support decisions based on practical and pragmatic outcomes.

Critical consciousness: What is it and what does it mean for students and practitioners?

Critical consciousness (CC) describes how oppressed or marginalized people learn to critically analyze their social conditions and act to change them (Watts *et al.*, 2011). For example, inequities in access to affordable healthcare, employment opportunities, and safe housing may pose barriers to an individual's performance within their daily occupational roles and inevitably their quality of life. Freire's CC theory is a philosophical, theoretical, and practice-based framework. It encompasses an individual's understanding of and action against the structural roots of personal and societal problems (e.g. low self-confidence, substance abuse, domestic violence, and racially motivated mass incarceration) (Freire, 1970).

The CC theory is an essential framework for occupational therapy students to understand and apply within the classroom and clinical learning spaces, as its relevance in addressing systematic inequities, promoting social justice, and advancing health equity is paramount for empowering and advocating for clients and in developing a therapeutic voice.

Here are ten key reasons why the CC theory is crucial for developing occupational therapy students, and some questions to prompt reflection on both academic and clinical learning spaces:

1. **Understanding structural inequities:** Critical conscience theory helps healthcare students recognize and understand the structural inequities embedded within healthcare systems and communities, including disparities in access to care, quality of care, and health outcomes. By critically examining the social, economic, and political determinants of health, students can identify root causes of health disparities and work toward action-based solutions that promote systematic change (Gregory *et al.*, 2022).

   - In comparison to the volitional choices by an individual (e.g. healthy eating, compliance to medical recommendations, lifestyle changes), can obesity also be related to having limited access to and affordance of nutritional foods and items, allocation of time and space for physical exercise, and awareness of health literacy for lifestyle changes to promote wellness outcomes?

2. **Recognizing implicit biases**: CC theory enables occupational therapy students to examine their own biases, assumptions, and privileges that may influence their interactions with clients from marginalized backgrounds (see Chapter 2). By fostering self-awareness and reflection, students can challenge implicit biases and

strive to provide equitable and culturally sensitive care to all patients, regardless of their race, ethnicity, gender, or socioeconomic status (Grenier, 2020).

- Are your perceptions of your classmates' access to health-related resources and experiences of health and wellness based on their gender, age, sexual orientation, cultural background(s), and/or wealth status?

3. **Promoting cultural competence:** CC theory emphasizes the importance of cultural competence in healthcare practice, encouraging students to understand, respect, and value the diverse cultural beliefs, values, and practices of their clients (see Chapter 5). By embracing cultural humility and engaging in opportunities to develop increased cultural humility and dialogue about cultural differences, occupational therapy students can enhance their abilities in establishing, improving, and sustaining the therapeutic trust and rapport that correlates to a greater degree of transparency within the occupational therapy process for all stakeholders.

- Is your awareness of other individuals' cultural backgrounds based on what you have been indirectly exposed to in your daily life (e.g. movies, social circles, general knowledge from online resources)? Do you believe this is a hindrance or a facilitator in how this knowledge shapes your biases about your cultural competence of other cultures, customs, and beliefs?

4. **Empowering those we serve:** CC theory empowers occupational therapy students to advocate for the rights and autonomy of their clients, particularly those from marginalized communities. By facilitating open communication, shared decision-making, and transparent therapeutic education, students can help empower clients to take an active role in their healthcare processes and advocate for their needs within healthcare systems (Hacker & Houry, 2022).

- What is your definition of marginalized communities? Is it based on implicit or explicit biases? Do you believe this perception has a negative or positive impact on the development of your clinical and critical reasoning skills within occupational therapy?

5. **Addressing SDOH:** CC emphasizes the importance of addressing SDOH, such as poverty, racism, housing instability, and food insecurity, which significantly impact health outcomes. Occupational therapy students can leverage their understanding of these social determinants to advocate for policies and interventions that address underlying systemic inequalities and promote health equity (Watts, 2011).

   - Do you believe that where a person lives and their type of dwelling have a direct correlation to the types of occupations they perform or can perform?

6. **Fostering health equity:** CC theory promotes a commitment to health equity, which involves ensuring that everyone has the opportunity to attain their highest level of health. By critically examining the distribution of resources, opportunities, and power within healthcare systems, students can identify disparities and advocate for policies and practices that promote equitable access to healthcare services and resources (Windsor *et al.*, 2022).

   - Do you believe that communities or neighborhoods with a higher index of wealth and resources equate to individuals with higher regard for their health and wellness and does this translate to generational knowledge?

7. **Advancing social justice:** CC theory aligns with principles of social justice, emphasizing the importance of challenging injustice, oppression, and discrimination within healthcare systems. Occupational therapy students can become agents of social change by advocating for policies and practices that dismantle systemic barriers to health equity and promote the well-being of marginalized populations.

   - Is social justice a form of occupational therapy intervention? Why or why not?

⊚ How does advancing social justice help us achieve the professional vision set by the American Occupational Therapy Association?

8. **Improving healthcare delivery:** CC theory can enhance the quality and effectiveness of healthcare delivery by encouraging students to critically evaluate existing systems and practices. By questioning traditional models of care, advocating for client-centered approaches, and incorporating principles of equity and social justice into their practice, students can contribute to more inclusive, responsive, and effective healthcare systems.

⊚ What steps can you take in relaying the meaning or benefit of advocating for social justice and self-advocacy to clients who come from cultural or ethnic backgrounds that do not recognize this belief/right/privilege?

9. **Enhancing interprofessional collaboration:** CC theory fosters collaboration and dialogue among healthcare professionals from diverse backgrounds, disciplines, and perspectives. By promoting mutual respect, understanding, and shared goals, students can work collaboratively to address complex health issues and advocate for comprehensive, interdisciplinary approaches to patient care and community health promotion (Hammell, 2015).

⊚ As an occupational therapy student, have you encountered dialogue or awareness from your peers within other healthcare sciences in relation to diversity, equity, inclusion, or other aspects of social justice issues (DEI+) (see Chapter 1) or advocacy? Why or why not?

10. **Preparing for future challenges:** In an increasingly diverse and complex healthcare landscape, CC theory equips occupational therapy students with the knowledge, skills, and mindset needed to navigate and address emerging challenges. By embracing a critical approach to healthcare practice, students can adapt to changing environments, advocate for marginalized communities, and

contribute to the advancement of health equity and social justice in the United States and beyond.

⊚ As an occupational therapy student, do you believe there will always be positive or automatic buy-in from individuals of marginalized backgrounds to take a lead in their own health and wellness outcomes? Why or why not?

CASE EXAMPLE 4.1: Malik and Christopher— "I feel as if we can relate, you know?"

During a group process course in which students are learning about the various types of group formats as a part of an intervention course, Malik and Christopher are paired together and start to practice an occupational profile from a case study example through simulated virtual software. The client they are both analyzing is of Indian descent and has deficits within their performance of daily activities due to pain experienced from a humeral fracture and an inability to afford time off from work. The simulated client also expresses feeling marginalized by his healthcare provider based on his accent. Malik makes fun of the simulation's accent by saying, "His accent is indeed funny, but I guess that's how the majority of them talk." Christopher is unsure of what Malik is referring to and asks, "What do you mean by the majority? Do you mean the accent or how they speak English? You know I'm Mexican and Haitian, Malik; we all don't sound the same, bro." Malik assumes that Christopher is a mixed-race individual who identifies with being Black first based on the complexion of his skin, and he quickly responds in a humorous tone, "Well, look at it this way, I guess just me, and Dr. Campbell, who know where we are truly from, don't we". Christopher is clearly confused by what Malik is insinuating and moves on from the conversation to complete their work within the allotted time before a class discussion is scheduled.

Reflective pause

- How would you describe the interaction between Christopher and Malik?
- Why do you think Dr. Campbell is mentioned by Malik in this exchange?

- What do you think Christopher is thinking when he is associated with an ethnic group based on the color of his skin?

Commentary on Case example 4.1
The interaction between Christopher and Malik can be viewed from a series of lenses that incorporate racism, stereotypes, biases, privilege, and general associations based on perceived racial identification. Although the conversation here is between two peers, it demonstrates how the sense of privilege can impact any component of an occupational therapy process. Occupational therapy students can reflect on how this interaction, if mirrored between a student and a client within a clinical learning space, may or may not negatively impact the therapeutic rapport and trust that are so critical to establishing and sustaining any therapeutic relationship. Using alternative strategies to foster space and time for discussion, could Christopher have approached Malik with a genuine need to understand where Malik was coming from when correlating Christopher's skin color to a perceived sense of privilege, in this case, a sense of belonging? Despite potentially feeling offended, could there be an opportunity to learn from this exchange that would highlight a greater degree of cultural humility and eventually build on competencies and sensitivities?

Recognizing factors related to privilege: Are accountability and ethics included?
Being aware of your own degree of privilege can be difficult for some and often a reflective process that takes a considerable amount of time, patience, and commitment. With an increasingly diversifying population, occupational therapy students are strategically advantaged in being trained and educated on integrating components of the social model of healthcare with the traditional scope of medical healthcare delivery. In essence, occupational therapy students are trained to not only analyze holistically how they can establish therapeutic gains for their clients, but also work on themselves to ensure that they are aware of their perceptions, biases, and privileges when advocating for the occupational rights of others through direct and indirect forms of services within any facet of the occupational therapy process. For example, the occupational profile can be a space where your sense of privilege can influence how implicit biases manifest into assumptions and beliefs within the therapeutic process.

Reflect on these questions

- Is health literacy a priority for all?
- Is technology literacy prioritized for all age groups?
- Is financial literacy a privilege for those with greater financial means than others?

Why is this a necessary point to understand from the lens of the occupational therapy student? Let's start from this angle first. If inequity is framed exclusively as a problem facing individuals who are "marginalized," then responses will only attempt to address the needs of these groups, without redressing the social structures causing this disadvantage (Dancy *et al.*, 2020; Brown & White, 2020). Unearned advantages or privileges compared to disadvantaged individuals (oppressed) are critical factors for any occupational therapy student to consider when understanding how occupations are formed, influenced, and adapted based on systematic enablers and disablers.

The Coin Model of Privilege and Critical Allyship (Nixon, 2019) embraces an intersectional approach to consider how systems of inequality, such as racism, heterosexism, and ableism, interact to produce complex patterns of unearned disadvantage and advantage (Nixon, 2019; Sharma *et al.*, 2018). For instance, one may consider the system of inequality of heterosexism. Heterosexism, a dominant norm in many societies, views being heterosexual as the norm, the de facto, the "right way" for sexual orientation. People who happen to fit this norm, because they are straight (i.e. heterosexual), enjoy advantages from this social structure. These advantages include openly expressing affection without fear of discrimination or violence—a privilege that may not be experienced by individuals of other sexual orientations. Heterosexuality is validated and valued through its regular, often positive, and default position as the "normal" way—a validation that is perpetuated in legal frameworks (i.e. laws and rights) and popular cinematic culture. Although benefiting from a society that accepts this normative lifestyle, heterosexuals did not earn this advantage; rather, they benefit from being societally accepted based on factors such as their culture, religion, geographic location, or sociopolitical climate. Other sexual orientations, on the other hand (e.g. homosexuality), may place individuals at a disadvantage (not an unearned advantage) merely because of the privilege bestowed by society on heterosexuality.

Table 1.4 describes some of the social groups that are typically associated with privilege in modern communities.

Table 4.1: Demographic and social characteristics and
the sense of privilege (Witten *et al.*, 2015; Yeager *et al.*, 2022)

Characteristics	Examples	Reflective considerations
Skin color	Brown	Does brown skin color automatically imply that the person is from an ethnic background?
Hair color/type	Black and natural	Does hair type imply ethnicity?
Cultural identity	Pacific Islander	Where are the Pacific Islands located?
Sexual orientation	Homosexual— gay	Why would this information be pertinent as part of a chart review for an occupational therapy student?
Gender	Female—straight	Why would this information be pertinent for a transgender occupational therapy provider?
Disability status	Disabled veteran	What does "disabled status" mean?
Mother's profession	Secretary	Does this contribute to the sense of privilege?
Father's profession	Custodian	Does this information contribute to the occupational therapy student's sense of bias?
Home location	Suburban	Does this information relate to privilege or socioeconomic status?
Home type	Apartment	Does any type of dwelling indicate a sense of impoverishment?
College attended	None	Why would this information be relevant to health literacy?
Languages spoken	Fluent in four languages	Is this information relevant for therapeutic rapport?
Employment status	Unemployed	Does this contribute to implicit bias?
Debt	None	Is this a form of privilege?

CASE EXAMPLE 4.2: Jamie talks to Dr. Campbell—"I don't understand what happened with Malik earlier this week"

It's been three days since Jamie spoke to Malik after their conversation when waking to school one morning and Jamie feels very upset. Jamie is not sure if she said something wrong or has offended Malik in any way and seeks out her faculty advisor for support. Jamie schedules a meeting with Dr. Campbell and discusses what happened. Jamie is not ready for what Dr. Campbell says during their meeting and it takes her by surprise. Dr. Campbell mentions terms such as "privilege," "sense of belonging," and "microaggressions" to Jamie and asked her to reflect on these points as she recollected what was said and occurred during that brief interaction with Malik earlier in the week. As a mediator, Dr. Campbell does not want to tell Jamie how or what to think but instead wants her to take this situation as a learning opportunity for self-growth, and highlights the importance of soft skills and emotional intelligence as critical interpersonal skills for the occupational therapy student and, most importantly, an opportunity for cultural humility.

Reflection pause

- What do you think Jamie is thinking about at that moment with Dr. Campbell?
- What would you say to Jamie after class?
- Do you think Jamie is insensitive in her interaction with Malik?
- If you relate to this incident, describe how you would react to Dr. Campbell's comments.
- Should Jamie speak to Malik directly?

Commentary on Case example 4.2

This example describes a deceivingly innocuous classroom exchange meant to encourage clinical reasoning and critical thinking skills. Faculty advisement or any form of valued mentorship is a useful opportunity for the occupational therapy student to engage in facilitated exploration, reflection, and safe and often private discussion of sensitive topics related to their academic areas of growth and development. This exchange between Jamie and Dr. Campbell highlights the importance of not solely seeking out answers but instead being prepared to delve into a period of self-analysis and introspection, skills often necessary within occupational therapy practice as forms of professional and personal development.

Let's think about it

A few days go by and Malik finally approaches Jamie at lunch and asks for a few minutes of her time. During their conversation, Malik expresses how uncomfortable he felt with Jamie's statement on buying breakfast, which implied that he could not afford it himself. He says that he does not think Jamie's comment was meant to be harmful or targeted in nature but it did trigger a feeling of inadequacy and of being judged for not having the same financial resources as her. Jamie during this situation is provided with a rare opportunity by Malik to reflect, ask questions, embrace humility, and take this as a learning platform, as opposed to feeling accused or attacked. Jamie expresses how thankful she is to Malik for creating this space to exchange their thoughts, beliefs, and experiences and how the concept of privilege could impact a social and therapeutic relationship in so many ways. Both Malik and Jamie display courage and growth during this exchange and many lessons are learned through creating this safe space for dialogue.

Recap

The interactions between Jamie and Malik, friends and peers of an occupational therapy program, are intended to introduce the multifaceted nature of the sense and awareness of privilege and how it not only can impact daily social interactions but also may influence any therapeutic process within occupational therapy education, practice, and research.

This scenario describes a critical moment of how privilege, biases, and critical consciousness can impact a therapeutic relationship for the developing occupational therapy student. This scenario is intended to allow the occupational therapy student to appreciate how a perceived sense of privilege or oppression can drastically shape the processes and outcomes of any personal and professional interaction, and the cognizant responsibility of the student to take into account their own biases and how they impact how our consumers feel and are judged, and how safe they feel around us.

Reflective thinking

- Do you think Jamie could apply what she has learned from this situation to a fieldwork experience?

Critical thinking

- Identify an inappropriate response by Malik during that initial exchange with Jamie that morning.

Action-oriented thinking

- Think of one action Malik can take in the *classroom* to address this experience (e.g. address this issue in a classroom conversation).
- Think of one action Jamie can take at the program level to address this experience (e.g. talk to the academic fieldwork coordinator)

HOT TAKE

In some cases, can people seek and attain privilege if they work hard enough? If so, why don't they?

Suggested reading to navigate this question: "Expanding the Definition of Privilege: The Concept of Social Privilege" (Black & Stone, 2005).

References

Black, L. L. & Stone, D. (2005). Expanding the definition of privilege: The concept of social privilege. *Journal of Multicultural Counseling and Development, 33*(4), 243–255. https://doi.org/10.1002/j.2161-1912.2005.tb00020.x

Brown, E. A. & White, B. M. (2020). Recognizing privilege as a social determinant of health during COVID-19. *Health Equity, 4*(1). http://doi.org/10.1089/heq.2020.0038

Dancy, M., Rainey, K., Stearns, E. *et al.* (2020). Undergraduates' awareness of White and male privilege in STEM. *International Journal of STEM Education, 7,* 52. https://doi.org/10.1186/s40594-020-00250-3

Doll, J., Malloy, J., & Gonzales, R. (2023). Social determinants of health: Critical consciousness as the core to collective impact. *Frontiers in Research Metrics and Analytics, 8,* 1141051. https://doi.org/10.3389/frma.2023.1141051

Freire, P. (1970). *Pedagogy of the Oppressed* (M.B. Ramos, Trans). Continuum.

Freire, P. (2020). "Pedagogy of the Oppressed." In *Toward a Sociology of Education* (pp.374–386). Routledge.

Gregory, A., White, B., & Brown, E. (2022). Examining privilege as a social determinant of health with undergraduate health care students. *Journal of Student Research, 11*(1). https://doi.org/10.47611/jsr.v11i1.1462

Grenier, M.-L. (2020). Cultural competency and the reproduction of White supremacy in occupational therapy education. *Health Education Journal, 79*(6), 633–644. https://doi.org/10.1177/0017896920902515

Hacker, K. & Houry, D. (2022). Social needs and social determinants: The role of the Centers for Disease Control and Prevention and Public Health. *Public Health Reports, 137*(6), 1049–1052. https://doi.org/10.1177/00333549221120244

Hacker, K., Auerbach, J., Ikeda, R., Philip, C., & Houry, D. (2022). Social determinants of health: An approach taken at CDC. *Journal of Public Health Management & Practice, 28*(6), 589–594. doi: 10.1097/PHH.0000000000001626

Hammell, K. R. W. (2015). Client-centred occupational therapy: The importance of critical perspectives. *Scandinavian Journal of Occupational Therapy, 22*(4), 237–243, doi: 10.3109/1 1038128.2015.1004103

Nixon, S. A. (2019). The coin model of privilege and critical allyship: Health implications. *BMC Public Health, 19*(1), 1637. https://doi.org/10.1186/s12889-019-7884-9

Sharma, M., Pinto, A. D., & Kumagai, A. K. (2018). Teaching the social determinants of health: A path to equity or a road to nowhere? *Academic Medicine, 93*(1), 25–30. doi: 10.1097/ ACM.0000000000001689

Watts, R. J., Diemer, M. A., & Voight, A. M. (2011). Critical consciousness: Current status and future directions. *New Directions for Child and Adolescent Development,* (134), 43–57. https:// doi.org/10.1002/cd.310

Windsor, L. C., Jemal, A., Goffnett, J., Smith, D. C., & Sarol Jr, J. (2022). Linking critical consciousness and health: The utility of the critical reflection about social determinants of health scale (CR_SDOH). *SSM—Population Health, 17,* 101034. https://doi.org/10.1016/j. ssmph.2022.101034

Witten, N. A. & Maskarinec, G. G. (2015). Privilege as a social determinant of health in medical education: A single class session can change privilege perspective. *Hawaii Journal of Medicine & Public Health, 74*(9), 297–301.

World Health Organization. (2025). *Social Determinants of Health.* www.who.int/health-topics/ social-determinants-of-health#tab=tab_1

Yeager, K. H., Gandara, G. A., & Martinez, C. (2022). "It's bigger than me:" Influence of social support on the development of self-advocacy for college students with disabilities. *Journal of Postsecondary Education and Disability, 35*(2), 145–159.

CHAPTER 5

Cultural Humility

"You always smell like curry!"

—————————— Razan Hamed PhD., OTR/L ——————————

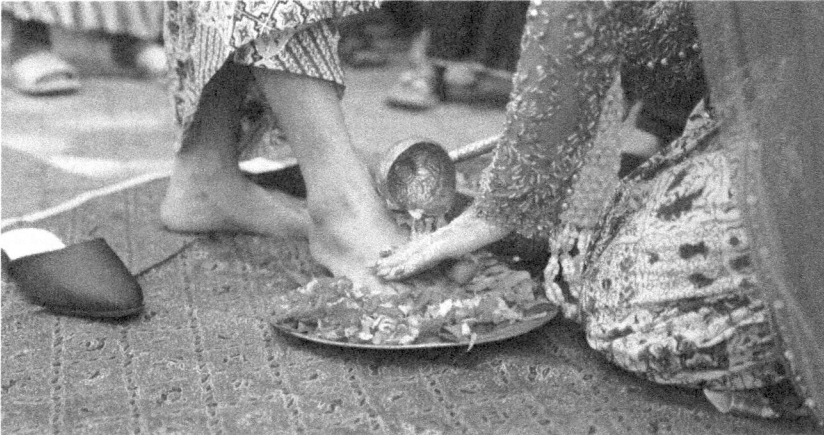

Chapter overview

In this chapter, we introduce cultural humility as an intentional mindset needed for ethical and inclusive practices within occupational therapy education and communities. Students can explore cases that challenge their critical thinking and present opportunities for growing into culturally intentional practitioners. We discuss the harmful effects of OT practices lacking cultural humility, and the power of cultural humility in OT education, practice, and interpersonal relationships. Students are invited to reflect on their understanding of the connection between DEI+ concepts and cultural humility throughout the chapter.

Content

- Cultural humility and other relevant terms.
- Cultural humility in the classroom, Case example 5.1: Merry Christmas!
- How community engagement enhances cultural humility, Case example 5.2: What is your neighborhood like?
- Cultural humility in fieldwork education, Case example 5.3: "Memona, you always smell like curry!"
- Cultural humility, privilege, and power, Case example 5.4: Let's talk about Mr. Jackson.
- Let's think about it.

Objectives

1. Identify the differences between cultural humility and other terms related to culture.
2. Describe behaviors and acts indicative of adequate or inadequate cultural humility.
3. Apply strategies to enhance a culturally humble mindset as a DEI+ mindful student.

Storyline snapshot

The students are starting their second year in their occupational therapy program. They continue to take courses together, working on group assignments, meeting with academic advisors, and attending various professional activities. Classroom conversations are a mix of new knowledge, personal and professional growth, and insight into issues within the world of DEI+. Other conversations are happening over meals, extracurricular activities while commuting, and at other campus corners. Regardless of where these conversations are happening, they are bringing another kind of growth—growth of the mind and self. Students are reflecting on their views of themselves, people, communities, and the world. These insights are not always pleasant but they are the steps that pave the way for bias-free spaces where everyone feels they belong.

In this chapter, Allie and Gemma are working on a clinical case study. By now, they have learned so much about each other except for the fact that they both have invisible disabilities affecting their daily activities.

An interesting conversation takes place about how culture and disability intersect and determine health outcomes. They later learn that making (or withholding) assumptions about one another can make all the difference in how the conversation ends.

Characters in this chapter (see the character matrix in Appendix 2 for details)

- Allie
- Gemma
- Memona
- Dr. Boyle
- Dr. Campbell
- Levi

Introduction

A lack of critical insight into professional knowledge increases the risk that occupational therapy will remain satisfied with the current understanding of culture, based on the dominant knowledge.

CASTRO ET AL., 2014, P.401

Occupational therapy practitioners (OTPs) work with individuals of different backgrounds, including age, gender, race, ethnicity, religion, ability, sexual orientation, and other human dimensions. Students and OTPs must recognize their preconceptions or implicit biases about a certain group to ensure an ethical and effective therapeutic relationship with all clients regardless of their backgrounds. Practitioners must always approach the interaction with openness and self-awareness to consider the power difference in the therapeutic relationship.

Power is the social advantage associated with real or perceived privilege conferred on a group of people due to race, ethnicity, or other attributes (Black & Stone, 2005). This process of reflecting on one's own biases while assessing the difference in privilege is called cultural humility (Tervalon & Murray-García, 1998). Cultural humility is a mindset, 'with which student practitioners continue to learn about the diversity of people across all human traits. This learning process also includes inspecting one's biases, understanding the concepts of social privilege and power, recognizing the complex nature of within-group diversity, and considering the sociopolitical climates affecting the client's and therapist's identities (see Chapter 4).

Cultural humility has been interchangeably used with terms such as cultural competence, cultural awareness, cultural sensitivity, and other similar phrases. Table 5.1 describes some of these definitions. Cultural humility is the most recently adopted term in social and healthcare sciences and is defined as a lifelong learning process when working with people of diverse cultural backgrounds and recognizing aspects of social privilege and power. Unlike other culture-centered terms, cultural humility emphasizes an unceasing process of learning, reflection, and appreciation of clients' diverse backgrounds regardless of the level of clinical experience (i.e. student, novice, or experienced OTP). Other terms described in Table 5.1 may not call for the same level of introspection (e.g. cultural awareness and sensitivity) or may assume that proficiency can be achieved with enough training (e.g. cultural competence) (Cross et al., 1989). Additionally, these terms assume that culture has a static and unchanging nature, with limited nuances among individuals within the same culture (Hammell, 2013).

Students must recognize the difference between cultural humility and cultural competence, given their common interchangeable use. While both terms call for critically inspecting one's biases and thinking about cultural differences among individuals, cultural humility emphasizes the diversity within groups and urges consideration of components of power. Unlike cultural competence, cultural humility does not warrant proficiency when working with diverse populations; instead, it calls for a lifelong obligation to learn about the dynamic nature of culture across various human sub-cultures (Agner, 2020).

Cultural humility calls for practitioners to intentionally recalibrate their mindset into one that fosters continuous reflections on daily communication with clients and other professionals. This "mindset reset" must take place while students are building their professional skills and before they plunge into clinical education or future practice (Govender et al., 2017). In fact, research shows that cultural humility does not come naturally with clinical practice and does not vary across clinical practice areas (Fedko et al., 2021), and it is recommended that students seek opportunities to build that skill throughout the occupational therapy program (Murden et al., 2008; Wittman & Velde, 2002).

Table 5.1: Terms related to cultural humility

Term	Description	Example
Cultural awareness	Mindfulness of culture as a construct affecting daily activities. Here there is little effort made to learn more about diverse cultures or the power dynamic between the therapist and the client. Limited emphasis on the need to recognize one's biases toward other cultures.	A student is *aware* of other cultures, ethnicities, and sexual orientations.
Cultural sensitivity	Awareness of diversity of cultures and recognizing the need to be responsive to cultural variations and delivering culturally relevant interventions. Yet limited emphasis on privilege, power, or biases.	A student *recognizes* that their classmates identify with different gender, racial, ethnic, religious, sexual, ability, and age groups.
Cultural competence	Gathering knowledge about various cultures while reflecting on one's own culture and biases (Awaad, 2003). Effort is made to learn about other cultures and the needs of clients of diverse backgrounds.	A faculty member *gathering* information about the Lunar Year celebration in the Asian culture.
Cultural humility	Constant learning-oriented process about the diversity of cultures and dynamic nature of privilege and health outcomes (Hammell, 2013).	An occupational therapy practitioner considers how meal preparation/eating is viewed and practiced in the client's culture (e.g. using group versus individual plates) and ensures *not to assume* that it is similar to the occupational therapy practitioner's culture. Additionally, the occupational therapy practitioner *asks and responds* to questions about meal time in a way that does not project their own biases on the client's cultural practice (e.g. refraining from saying "Interesting" or "That's different").
Cultural safety	Considering the intersection of cultural, political, and social aspects with healthcare disparities when treating marginalized people (the term was created around indigenous people of New Zealand (Polaschek, 1998)	Considering how legal citizenship status affects access to quality healthcare and health literacy in patients with undocumented immigration conditions.

Note: The terms defined in this table are common at the time of writing this chapter. New terms emerge to reflect new realities and sociopolitical contexts.

Cultural humility in the classroom

Applying a cultural humility mindset is not exclusive to clinical practice. It is an approach that challenges the students to employ their critical thinking skills throughout the learning process. Students can think about how their social privilege (i.e. power) affects their academic outcomes, health, and professional well-being as learners. Additionally, students must recognize their "positioning" or "social location" on the privilege continuum that is typically associated with aspects of power that are related to race, gender, ability, sexuality, religion, and other diversity dimensions (Hammell, 2013, p.226). For example, a student who identifies with a marginalized community, speaks English as a second language, has a disability, has limited financial resources, or identifies as a first-generation learner is already positioned to face several academic disparities compared to a student who is privileged in these areas. Being aware of one's advantaged social position triggers self-reflection on how we interact with others in our occupation areas. When students are aware of the impact of their positioning they are better equipped to self-advocate and to seek support when and if needed to optimize occupational opportunities (i.e. critical consciousness, see Chapter 4). Failure to recognize the impact of positioning and social privilege may inadvertently elicit self-doubt, stress, and internalized inadequacy, which may eventually lead to poor academic outcomes and well-being.

Students must also be aware of their daily interactions with faculty and students of different statuses of power and privilege. The social identity wheel (see Chapter 3) is a good example of how to reflect on one's own and others' identities and how they may facilitate or limit access to occupational opportunities (e.g. ability to work as a teaching assistant), intended outcomes (e.g. better grades), or self-concept (e.g. feeling inadequate). Therefore, a mindset of cultural humility is important not only to recognize our own culture and biases and those of others but also to recognize how others interact with us based on our own cultures. This awareness can help us identify signs of bias and microaggressions inflicted by others in the classroom.

CASE EXAMPLE 5.1: Merry Christmas!

Dr. Boyle is giving a class in the Fall semester on community-based interventions for first-year entry-level doctoral students at a suburban private university. She describes an assignment for a local nursing home in preparation for their capstone presentations. A student asks for suggestions for the assignment that have been successful in past years. Dr. Boyle states, "Think of the local communities and what matters to them at this time. For example, we are a few weeks away from Christmas—Merry Christmas by the way—a great activity would be to decorate a tree, wrap gifts, and prepare Christmas dinners and other popular activities for the season. Of course, whatever other holidays you can think of can count for the assignment too."

Reflective pause

- What do you think of the suggestion Dr. Boyle makes during class? Think of choosing Christmas as a default holiday.
- How can Dr. Boyle model cultural humility using the same example? Think of a different wording or phrasing for her suggestion.
- Do you think Dr. Boyle is culturally mindful when she says, "...whatever other holidays"?

Commentary on Case example 5.1

The scenario describes an example of an activity that may indeed be relevant for many people who celebrate Christmas, including students. Although Dr. Boyle does allude to exploring other holidays celebrated during the season, the phrase "whatever other holidays you can think of" implies that these holidays are not as central to the community as Christmas. This default Christianity is one example that can make students in that classroom who celebrate other holidays feel "othered" and marginalized. A better option for Dr. Boyle could be for her to ask the students the question: "What holidays do you think would be relevant for this local nursing home?" This alternative phrasing provides the students with an opportunity to highlight their own cultures or shed light on diversity within each culture (e.g. Christians who may not celebrate Christmas).

Cultural humility and community engagement

Depending on what groups the students identify with within their communities, local, national, or global events can affect students' occupations. Recognizing the social movements and economic, sociopolitical, and theoretical issues affecting occupation across diverse groups of people in the community is a key component of cultural humility (Castro *et al.*, 2014). Additionally, students interact with community-dwelling persons, groups, and populations who are also impacted by the events and conditions of their communities. Being informed about how events in the community affect daily function increases the students' and practitioners' insight into components of power and privilege, which is necessary for a cultural humility approach. This level of awareness is unlikely to be achieved by merely learning about cultural humility in the classroom or going through formal training on cultural humility (Shepherd, 2019). Engaging in various levels of communities (see the Macro-Micro Model of Diversity in Chapter 3) will enhance students' awareness of the intersection between the community and the individual. Examples include following the local news on current events, volunteering, and attending advocacy events by state and national OT associations.

Students can also bring awareness to these issues in the classroom by highlighting experiences within their communities if they feel comfortable doing so. For example, students can recognize in-class cultural events that may not usually receive media attention (e.g. religious holidays). Additionally, students may be impacted by disturbances that are instigated by bias and prejudice, such as racially based hate crimes, anti-semitism, Islamophobia, homophobia, ableism, bullying, and other hate-based incidents. Faculty members can play a key role in creating spaces for students that facilitate such engagement.

CASE EXAMPLE 5.2: What is your neighborhood like?

Dr. Campbell is running a class on social determinants of health, and invites the students to reflect on the overturn of the Roe versus Wade case by the Supreme Court on June 24, 2022. She states, "How does this decision affect the daily occupations of women of marginalized communities compared to women with privilege, or women with lower rather than higher socioeconomic status?" The prompt stirs an interesting discussion in class, with many students sharing their perspectives. Memona responds to the question by highlighting the prohibition of abortion in Islam and as this is a marginalized group of women, the Supreme Court decision may not affect Muslims the same way that it does other marginalized communities. Levi highlights the nature of the issue for transgender women and explains that it may be complicated due to the current legislation around gender-affirming care. Gemma highlights multiple layers of issues affecting Afro-Latina women, including the socioeconomic burden and the stigma of being a single parent, as well as limited childcare available for working mothers on single incomes. Dr. Campbell invites the rest of the class to discuss in pairs the information they have heard from their classmates and identify a follow-up question.

Reflective pause

- If you were sitting in that class, what aspects would you address to answer Dr. Campbell's question?
- Do any of the perspectives shared by the students in the scenario surprise you? Explain why or why not.
- What is the value of having the students come up with a follow-up question?

Commentary on Case example 5.2

The scenario describes how cultural humility can be fostered in the classroom by inviting students to share how events directly or indirectly affect members of their communities. Dr. Campbell creates an opportunity for the students to bring their perspectives to the discussion. Students highlight different aspects of the same issue based on the lived experiences of women from their communities. This perspective is almost impossible to be taught to students via readings or classroom activities alone. Even students who do not engage in the discussion are invited to reflect on the information they have received and identify a follow-up question as a means for reflection. Questions encourage students to reflect on the topic of discussion, which if facilitated properly can foster culturally mindful conversations.

Cultural humility in fieldwork education and clinical practice

Students take the first steps toward clinical practice through fieldwork education. During this clinical portion of the OT curriculum, students either observe or work with clients, caregivers, and other professionals in various practice settings. Practicing cultural humility prepares students to work with individuals of diverse backgrounds in a client-centered approach. This includes navigating the OT process through a lens of human diversity when gathering information about daily activities, selecting culturally tailored assessment tools, and planning culturally appropriate interventions. A lack of cultural humility can negatively affect the outcomes of any treatment plan in healthcare (Shepherd, 2019), especially for clients of marginalized communities.

A culturally mindful therapist ensures that the intervention plan is informed by the client's cultural norms, beliefs, and preferences even for the most basic components of the OT process (e.g. independence). For example, a therapist's perception of what functional independence looks like in daily activities (based on what they learn in OT school) may affect all subsequent steps in intervention planning and implementation for a particular client. Some cultures value co-independence (i.e. a group or family-oriented norm that involves other caregivers in completing daily activities regardless of the level of individual independence) over individual independence (e.g. completing activities without involving others in activity completion). The outcomes of this process may not align with the client's goals if the client's desired level of independence is different from the therapist's perception (e.g. individual independence versus co-independence).

> **CASE EXAMPLE 5.3: "Memona, you always smell like curry!"**
> Memona is an MOT (Master-level OT student) student in the first Fieldwork II rotation in the inpatient rehabilitation unit and is currently under the direct supervision of the OT fieldwork educator (FWE) on site. During the lunch break, the supervisor talks with Memona about the morning session and shares some feedback about Memona's performance. The conversation is positive yet strictly professional and communication is clear, with no issues. The FWE then ends the conversation with this statement: "Oh, before I forget. I hope I am not being offensive because I really do not mean to, but a couple of colleagues pointed out that it always smells like curry when you are around. Although I don't mind it, it may trigger some breathing issues for some patients. Just something to think about."

Reflective pause

- What do you think of the FWE's comment about Memona's smell? Is it culturally appropriate?

- Can you think of an alternative way of speaking to Memona about the smell?
- Do you think Memona would (or should) be offended or upset about the comment?
- How do you think Memona should respond to that comment?

Commentary on Case example 5.3

The scenario describes an interaction between an FWE and a student in a busy hospital setting. The FWE has a supervisory role over Memona, which implies a power dynamic of controlling Memona's performance evaluation and eventually her passing grade. Memona, like other students during a fieldwork rotation, needs to pass the fieldwork requirement to proceed in the program. Students are expected to effectively communicate with the FWE to improve clinical and professional performance and eventually pass the fieldwork requirements. The scenario reflects a positive professional interaction up to the point where the FWE makes the comments about the smell. Although the reason behind the feedback is clear and may be reasonable to some extent, the comment dismisses the power dynamic inherent in this interaction, with Memona having no choice whether or not to agree to this portion of the feedback. A power-mindful approach is recommended where the FWE prefaces the statement by saying, "Do you mind if I make a suggestion that is not related to your clinical performance per se but something you may be interested to be aware of or to think about" or, "I have some feedback that I received from other people working with you. Do you mind if I share it?" This alternative wording may prepare Memona to receive likely unpleasant feedback and enable her to ask clarifying questions. It is also important for the FWE to highlight that this is not directly related to Memona's performance and hence will not affect her evaluation outcomes. This mitigates any anxiety that may be caused by this comment. Additionally, it is important for the FWE to allow Memona the opportunity to respond to this comment, whether at the moment or later in the week.

Cultural humility, privilege, and intersectionality

OT students must understand the concepts of power and privilege to practice cultural humility in any daily interactions. Historically, social privilege was linked to the social construct of gender and race, where women and people of color were most likely to be affected by injustices (e.g. gender-based pay inequality or housing) and oppression (i.e. explicit discrimination). Oppressed social groups had less access to life opportunities such as good education, healthcare services, health literacy, and employment. Limited access to these opportunities is associated with poor life and health outcomes (Robinson, 1999). Power is linked to social privilege. In this context, power is defined as the naturally granted access to advantages and opportunities solely due to one's inclusion in a certain social category (e.g. being born White or cis-male). The concepts of power and privilege were extended to include other social categories such as age, faith, socioeconomic status, sexual orientation, and ability (Black & Stone, 2005). Additionally, these concepts expanded to consider the intersectionality of social groups and their effect on favorable life opportunities, such as academic success and employment (Crenshaw, 2019).

Therefore, the social groups a client identifies with and their intersectionality may determine privileged access to quality education, healthcare, vocations, social status, and other areas of occupation. Practicing cultural humility urges students and practitioners to consider privilege and power when treating individuals of various backgrounds. This means considering the factors that may have contributed to the current and future status of functional independence. For example, a client with limited healthcare coverage or insurance may not have access to OT services, technology, telehealth, equipment, or even time to improve their health outcomes. Therefore, as part of being culturally mindful, one must explore all the determinants of functional independence while planning therapeutic interventions (e.g. while completing an occupational profile in fieldwork education).

CASE EXAMPLE 5.4: Let's talk about Mr. Jackson

Allie and Gemma are working together on a case study (Mr. Jackson) for a course on physical dysfunction. Mr. Jackson is a 54-year-old Black Hispanic male with type II diabetes and hypertension. He is currently being fitted for an above-knee prosthetic post-amputation. The students are required to complete an occupational profile where they identify potentially affected occupation areas and client factors that must be explored when completing the occupational profile.

While completing the assignment Allie makes the following

comment: "It breaks my heart when I see amputation cases after diabetes because I feel this is a totally preventable cause of disability. It is like something within our control, you know." Gemma responds with, "Maybe" to Allie's comment. Allie exclaims "Maybe?! Why, you don't think so? Listen, I know what disabilities feel like, especially when you can't prevent or control them. So diabetes sounds like something you can control by making better daily choices."

Gemma pauses for a second and then responds, "I am not sure this is fair. I mean, I don't know how much you know about diabetes, to be honest, but not all people have choices. Sometimes they just don't know any better, and sometimes there is actually nothing you can do about it." Allie then responds, "I am dyslexic, a disability I can't control, and there isn't a lifestyle I can change to fix it but if I had diabetes, I would have done something about it."

Gemma then responds, "Well, I am type I diabetic and there are not any life choices I could have made to prevent it. As a matter of fact, it took my parents a while to figure out what is wrong with me... and I am sorry you have dyslexia."

Allie says, "I am so sorry that you're diabetic. I didn't know."

Reflective pause

- Do you agree with Allie's comment? Is it a sign of empathy or a lack of cultural humility?
- Why do you think Gemma does not fully agree with Allie's remark? Consider Gemma's social groups.
- If you were part of this conversation, how would you respond to Allie's comment? Consider privilege and power.
- What aspects of Mr. Jackson's social identity or intersectionality should Gemma and Allie be exploring?

Commentary on Case example 5.4

The scenario describes a casual conversation between two classmates working on a case study. Mr. Jackson identifies with a historically marginalized social group, with limited access to quality health education or healthcare. Although Allie's comment does reflect a sense of empathy with Mr. Jackson, it carries an assumption that Mr. Jackson's disability could have been prevented had he chosen a more mindful lifestyle.

While this may be true in some cases in terms of daily habits, cultural humility requires us to explore all aspects of our social identities and how they may have led to current health and functional outcomes. Allie may not intend to be presumptuous of Mr. Jackson's lifestyle of health habits, but her comments indicate limited exposure to these marginalized communities and social determinants of health (i.e. factors related to social identities that affect health outcomes). Gemma being of a similar social group may have a perception of how this social group may face determinants of health and function that are not necessarily controllable. A more culturally humble approach Allie can take in the future is to consider how health outcomes can be associated with social privilege (or the lack thereof) when collecting information about patients.

Let's think about it

Social privilege means that members of a certain social group may have access to advantages or opportunities for better health or life outcomes. But it also means that a member of that group may not be aware of the life experiences of less previewed groups. This means that members of that privileged group may not be cognizant of what factors may have led to certain unfavorable health outcomes such as disability, poor education, limited health and technology literacy, and lack of financial stability. Allie represents many members of privileged communities who may be unaware of the social determinants of health of someone like Mr. Jackson. While being unaware is not the problem, making assumptions about a person or a social group may affect our judgment and decision-making for a client's care. Historically, marginalized communities with limited privilege were perceived to be responsible for being unprivileged due to a lack of "trying" (Black & Stone, 2005).

A productive approach of cultural humility will urge the individual to actively and intentionally learn about the marginalized community and how social determinants of health exist in our communities. Pursuing information, refraining from making assumptions, and asking non-judgmental questions are some of the things people can do to learn more about the interplay between privilege and health.

Although unintended, the comment made by Allie may be triggering for Gemma since she may have relatable experiences to Mr. Jackson. What happens next in that conversation is shaped by Allie's innocuous comment and assumption about Mr. Jackson. For example, Gemma may choose to share information with Allie about the Hispanic/Latino/LatinX community, including historical contexts of colonization, immigration practices in the US, healthcare coverage, and ethnic traumas to name a few. Alternatively, Gemma may also choose to say nothing and opt to ignore Allie's clarifying question. Either way, Gemma's decision is a pivotal point in that conversation on cultural humility. The scenario also shows the harmful effect of making assumptions about someone's life choices, cultures, and abilities based on their backgrounds.

Reflective thinking

- How do you think Gemma should respond to Allie's question?
- While reflecting on your social privilege how would you respond or perceive Allie's comment?
- Which character do you empathize with the most? Why?

Critical thinking

- Can Allie's comment be perceived as a microaggression (see Chapter 3)?
- Should Gemma seek clarifying information from Allie so as not to misjudge her question?

Action-oriented thinking

- How would you engage the fieldwork educator in this conversation?
- What resources would you recommend in this scenario to make it culturally informed?

HOT TAKE

How can cultural humility be the pathway to dismantling oppression, racism, and White supremacy?

Suggested reading to navigate this question: "Cultural competency and the reproduction of White supremacy in occupational therapy education" (Grenier, 2020).

References

Agner, J. (2020). Moving From cultural competence to cultural humility in occupational therapy: A paradigm shift. *American Journal of Occupational Therapy, 74*(4), 7404347010p1–7404347010p7. https://doi.org/10.5014/ajot.2020.038067

Awaad, J. (2003). Culture, cultural competency, and occupational therapy: A review of the literature. *British Journal of Occupational Therapy, 66*(8), 356–362. https://doi.org/10.1177/030802260306600804

Black, L. L. & Stone, D. (2005). Expanding the definition of privilege: The concept of social privilege. *Journal of Multicultural Counseling and Development, 33*(4), 243–255. https://doi.org/10.1002/j.2161-1912.2005.tb00020.x

Castro, D., Dahlin-Ivanoff, S., & Mårtensson, L. (2014). Occupational therapy and culture: A literature review. *Scandinavian Journal of Occupational Therapy, 21*(6), 401–414. https://doi.org/10.3109/11038128.2014.898086

Crenshaw, K. (2019). *On Intersectionality: Essential Writings.* New Press.

Cross, T. L., Bazron, B. J., Dennis, K. W., & Isaacs, M. R. (1989). *Towards a Culturally Competent System of Care: Volume 1.* Georgetown University Child Development Center.

Fedko, S. L., Kurbatova, A., Remesnyk, N., Matviienko, I., *et al.* (2021). Cultural awareness in contemporary mental health practice. *Wiadomości Lekarskie, 74*(11), 2762–2767. https://doi.org/10.36740/WLek202111114

Govender, P., Mpanza, D. M., Carey, T., Jiyane, K., Andrews, B., & Mashele, S. (2017). Exploring cultural competence amongst OT students. *Occupational Therapy International,* 1–8. https://doi.org/10.1155/2017/2179781

Grenier, M. L. (2020). Cultural competency and the reproduction of White supremacy in occupational therapy education. *Health Education Journal, 79*(6), Article 6. https://doi.org/10.1177/0017896920902515

Hammell, K. R. (2013). Occupation, well-being, and culture: Theory and cultural humility. *Canadian Journal of Occupational Therapy, 80*(4), Article 4. https://doi.org/10.1177/0008417413500465

Murden, R., Norman, A., Ross, J., Sturdivant, E., Kedia, M., & Shah, S. (2008). Occupational therapy students' perceptions of their cultural awareness and competency. *Occupational Therapy International, 15*(3), 191–203. https://doi.org/10.1002/oti.253

Polaschek, B. A. (1998). Cultural safety: A new concept in nursing people of different ethnicities. *Journal of Advanced Nursing, 27*(3), 452–457. https://doi.org/10.1046/j.1365-2648.1998.00547.x

Robinson, T. L. (1999). The Intersections of dominant discourses across race, gender, and other identities. *Journal of Counseling & Development, 77*(1), 73–79. https://doi.org/10.1002/j.1556-6676.1999.tb02423.x

Shepherd, S. M. (2019). Cultural awareness workshops: Limitations and practical consequences. *BMC Medical Education, 19*(1), 14. https://doi.org/10.1186/s12909-018-1450-5

Tervalon, M. & Murray-García, J. (1998). Cultural humility versus cultural competence: A critical distinction in defining physician training outcomes in multicultural education. *Journal of Health Care for the Poor and Underserved, 9*(2), 117–125. https://doi.org/10.1353/hpu.2010.0233

Wittman, P. & Velde, B. P. (2002). Attaining cultural competence, critical thinking, and intellectual development: A challenge for occupational therapists. *American Journal of Occupational Therapy, 56*(4), 454–456. https://doi.org/10.5014/ajot.56.4.454

CHAPTER 6

Empathy and Professionalism

"What's the big deal, Dr. Taylor?"

——— Vikram Pagpatan EdD, OTR/L, FAOTA ———

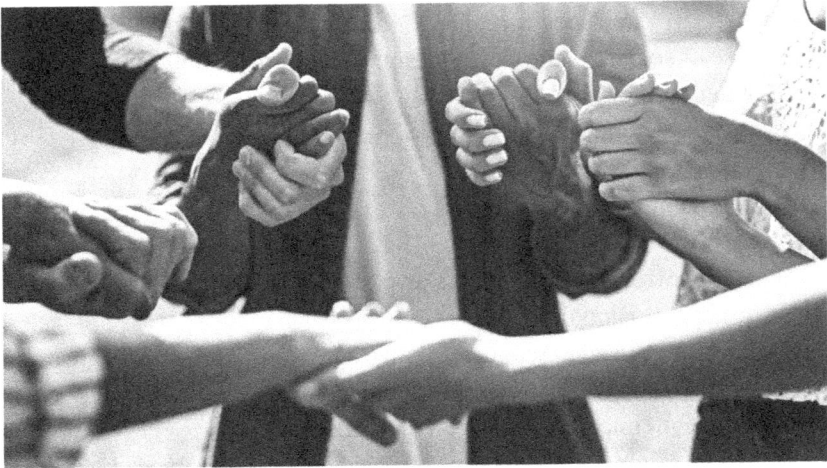

Chapter overview

The discussion of empathy within occupational therapy education and practice serves as a critical facilitator for students to grow into their clinical roles and for clinicians to adhere to the profession's code of ethics. The purpose of this chapter is to introduce the occupational therapy student to the various components of empathy, opportunities to reflect on the differences between empathy and other interpersonal skills, and why developing empathy authentically through reflective and experiential forms of learning is paramount to practicing a truly client-centered approach. Further, the chapter will discuss how empathy is necessary not only in clinical practice but also in other facets of professionalism within personal and digital contexts. We connect empathy to e-professionalism and digital citizenship such as online communication, electronic learning, and social media. Opportunities to reflect on the role of empathy in addressing issues related to diversity, equity, inclusion, and other aspects of social justice (DEI+) are provided throughout the chapter.

Content

- Empathy in occupational therapy: why does it matter?
- Empathy, sympathy, and clinical empathy, Case example 6.1: Jennie and Elizabeth—"What's the big deal?"
- Empathy, professionalism, and e-professionalism.
- Empathy and accountability, and digital citizenship: DEI+ and the use of social media, Case example 6.2: Jennie, Malik, and Christopher are not getting along.
- Let's think about it.

Objectives

1. Recognize basic constructs and terminology related to empathy and professionalism.
2. Identify the significance of empathy in personal communication and in embracing the development of professional intelligence in OT academic and clinical environments.
3. Apply strategies to navigate learning experiences in academic and clinical environments as related to the use of empathetic skills and professional intelligence.

Storyline snapshot

"It's time for good old neuro jeopardy!" shouts Dr. Taylor as xe starts class early on a Thursday morning. Dr. Taylor is well known for xyr humorous and engaging style of teaching, especially with difficult concepts, as xe is an avid believer in emphasizing neurological conditions and their impact on daily occupations. Dr. Taylor teaches a joint module (master's and doctoral students together). Although the class has begun, Jennie and Elizabeth are running late after a long study session the night before. They both walk in nearly 20 minutes after the start of the class. As the class resumes, Dr. Taylor shows video clips of pediatric clients with neuromotor conditions engaging in play and the class is asked to reflect in small groups. Jennie expresses to Malik and Christopher that she feels sad for the parents of that child and what they must be going through raising a child with such severe disabilities. Malik and Christopher also express similar sentiments but also discuss how play may be impacted due to a lack of voluntary mobility. Christopher mentions how he has heard of adaptive toys that may be a good fit, to which Malik responds with suggestions from their assistive technology class. After a few days, Jennie and Elizabeth both received an email from Dr. Taylor stating that their lateness on Thursday was never followed up with formal communication and that they have both lost half a letter grade toward their final examination.

Characters in this chapter (see character matrix in Appendix 2 for details)

- Dr. Taylor
- Malik
- Christopher
- Elizabeth
- Jennie

Introduction

I think we all have empathy. We may not have enough courage to display it.

MAYA ANGELOU

Consider a time within your academic and clinical journey when empathy served as a basis for connecting with others on a level that fostered a deeper therapeutic relationship. For example, if you met a classmate who shared your race, ethnicity, spoken language, faith, ability status, sexual orientation, or even the love for pets! That connection may have persisted throughout your time on the occupational therapy program or even flourished into your future role as a practitioner. The absence of empathy, on the other hand, may have limited the opportunities for connecting with other classmates, instructors, or even future clients. Empathy is key in building or demolishing human interaction and can impact all forms of communication, whether this is personal, professional, or digital.

The value of empathy within healthcare education has been widely researched (Boyleo *et al.*, 2018; King & Holosko, 2011; MacFarlane *et al.*, 2017), with an increasing body of literature distinguishing empathy from sympathy within the context of medical sciences (McNulty & Politis, 2023; Stanley *et al.*, 2020; Winter *et al.*, 2020). However, research examining the impact of teaching empathy in medical education and future clinical practice is still limited (Samarasekera *et al.*, 2023). Although being highly empathetic is not a standing requisite skill for occupational therapy practitioners (OTPs), employing empathy in clinical practice is key for establishing rapport in the therapeutic process. Understanding the impact of empathy within academic and clinical spaces requires entuned observational skills and a variety of interpersonal traits that allow the student and practitioner to venture beyond the disease or disability process and connect to the impact on everyday life. For instance, within fieldwork, actively listening coupled with reflection is an important skill to employ within both clinical and non-clinical situations, especially when using non-verbal gestures to express empathy beyond just spoken language. Empathy is a term widely used in social and medical sciences but was first defined in the social psychology domain as the capacity to think and feel oneself into the inner life of another person (Rogers, 1975).

In this chapter, we discuss how DEI+, empathy, professionalism, and digital citizenship are connected and can relate to the occupational therapy profession's code of ethics.

Empathy, sympathy, and clinical empathy

From a healthcare model, empathy has shifted from a social or interpersonal skill to a cognitive process in which aspects of affect, imagination or conceptualization, behavior, and reflection are embraced as processes to achieve an empathetic state (Irving & Dickson, 2004). This is where empathy and sympathy are commonly used interchangeably, despite the critical difference between the two terms.

Empathy versus sympathy and DEI+ issues

Empathy is when you consider your lived experiences as a story in which you have experienced opportunities to embrace empathy as a means of connecting, analyzing, and feeling a sense of belonging within situations that are often hard to understand from a human level. Hence, empathy is not only the identification but also the awareness of one's separateness from the observed action/emotion/behavior (Aring, 1958). This is critical for occupational therapy students as future practitioners in establishing strong therapeutic relationships (e.g. brainstorming ideas to enhance the daily functioning of a child with severe physical disabilities). Empathy is also necessary for addressing issues related to DEI+, and lack of empathy is the root of implicit bias, microaggressions, and ableism. For example, if you share a trait with another person (e.g. both diagnosed with a mental health condition) then you are more likely to relate to and understand the daily experiences of that person (e.g. stigma, the emotional burden, and the impact on daily functioning) and empathy will better help you support or advocate for them, knowing the difficult experiences they are going through. Inevitably, employing a sense of empathy can enhance a sense of belonging to other people in our communities, especially those of marginalized and unprivileged communities.

Sympathy, on the other hand, is the capacity for or act of entering into or sharing the feelings of another person, group, or community. This phenomenon is emotional and does not involve separating one's experience from others, which may eventually lead to emotional burnout (e.g. crying over seeing a child with severe physical disabilities). Showing sympathy for someone is not equivalent to empathy as it may not warrant supporting or advocating for that person, given the emotional (rather than the analytical) nature of sympathy.

Clinical empathy

Empathy is key to establishing therapeutic relationships with our clients. However, occupational therapy students (who transition into future clinicians) are most likely to employ a more practical form of empathy that can be used within practice called *clinical empathy*, which is predominantly a cognitive attribute combined with a capacity to communicate this understanding (Berger, 1987). Clinical empathy is defined as predominantly *cognitive as opposed to affective or emotional*, an attribute that entails an understanding, as opposed to a feeling, of the client's pain and suffering, combined with a capacity to communicate or translate this understanding and an intention to help through an outcome-focused model of care (Hojat *et al.*, 2020; Hojat *et al.*, 2018).

Since traditional empathy also entails an affective component, the rate of burnout and blurring of personal and professional boundaries have been examined and found to compromise client safety and processes that protect both the provider and clients (Tan *et al.*, 2020). The occupational therapy student will experience instances where sympathy and empathy are difficult to distinguish as both observable and exhibited emotions and behaviors; however, as a learner, these instances of blurred lines between both skills can also serve as opportunities for growth and reflection. Simply stated, occupational therapy students must experience opportunities to embrace both sympathy and empathy to understand which can be leveraged clinically to foster a deeper therapeutic relationship with those they serve within the profession.

Table 6.1 shows ten strategies in which an occupational therapy student can employ clinical empathy over sympathy and empathy.

Table 6.1: Ten strategies for employing clinical empathy

Strategies	Description	Examples
Active listening	Practice active listening skills by fully focusing on what patients are saying, without interrupting or jumping to conclusions.	This requires a form of comprehension that can be exhibited or conveyed to respective consumers, which may include clients, family members, other professionals and staff as well as clinical educators. How can you demonstrate your comprehension of what you have actively listened to?
Non-verbal communication	Pay attention to non-verbal cues such as body language and facial expressions to better understand patients' emotions and concerns.	This includes your tone, body language, and even cultural aspects of how you demonstrate your acknowledgment, presence, and authentication of the experiences shared between peers, faculty, and clients.
Empathetic language	Use empathetic language to convey understanding and support, such as acknowledging patients' feelings and validating their experiences.	Consider actions that you feel demonstrate the differences between sympathy and empathy within everyday situations. Now transform that skill to how you would exhibit clinical empathy within a clinical learning space.

Cultural humility	Develop cultural competence to understand and respect the diverse backgrounds and beliefs of patients, which can enhance empathy and communication.	Do you believe cultural competence is a static or dynamic process within occupational therapy education and practice?
Putting yourself in their shoes	Actively try to imagine what it would be like to be in the patient's situation, considering their perspective and feelings.	How can you authentically embody this reflection? What could you do as an occupational therapy student to foster a deeper appreciation of the empathetic state within occupational therapy education and practice?
Building rapport	Establish a rapport with patients to create a supportive environment where they feel comfortable expressing themselves openly.	What do you believe would happen if you were not able to establish or maintain rapport with a client within fieldwork?
Emotional regulation	Practice emotional regulation techniques to manage your own emotions effectively, allowing you to stay calm and empathetic in challenging situations.	Do you believe certain occupational therapy practice areas make it more difficult to regulate your emotions?
Respecting autonomy	Respect patients' autonomy by involving them in decision-making processes and honoring their preferences and values.	Why is autonomy within the profession's code of ethics?
Follow-up and continuity of care	Demonstrate empathy by following up with patients and providing continuity of care, showing that you are invested in their well-being beyond immediate interactions.	How can you demonstrate your investment in the therapeutic process within practice without crossing the personal–professional boundary?
Self-reflection and feedback	Regularly reflect on your interactions with patients and seek feedback from peers and mentors to continually improve your empathetic communication skills.	Why is self-reflection a critical part of occupational therapy education?

CASE EXAMPLE 6.1: Jennie and Elizabeth— "What's the big deal?"

Jennie and Elizabeth are utterly confused and upset after receiving an email from Dr. Taylor about arriving late to class earlier this week. Jennie is communicating with Elizabeth via text messaging and states,

"What's the big deal?" Elizabeth has greater awareness of why Dr. Taylor has emailed this communication and recalls a statement earlier in the semester in which Dr. Taylor informed the class, "Treat every class as if you are managing a rehabilitation clinic, and consider what types of attributes you would expect in your staff." This statement resonates with Elizabeth, who understands where Dr. Taylor is coming from; however, Jennie continues to feel distraught and conveys her emotions on social media by posting a statement on her public account, stating, "There are certain professors this semester who need to take a chill pill." Elizabeth decides to request a meeting with Dr. Taylor to further discuss the incident, but Jennie refuses the invitation extended by Elizabeth.

Reflective pause

- How would you describe the reactionary differences between Jennie and Elizabeth?
- Do you believe Dr. Taylor is justified in xyr actions?
- Is Jennie justified in making that statement on her public social media platform?

Commentary on Case example 6.1

Both Jennie and Elizabeth react very differently to Dr. Taylor's email. Whether emotions are at play or there are clear violations of communication, confidentiality, or transparency, the actions of Jennie and Elizabeth both reflect two spectrums of empathy and professionalism. The accountability of using social media platforms as an occupational therapy student also correlates to whether there are clear boundaries between the personal persona of the occupational therapy student and the developing professional identity. In turn, you must reflect and consider whether Jennie is justified in stating her comment within her personal social media platform which is also publicly accessible, and how this action may or may not reflect on any professional code of conduct/integrity and/or ethical standards not only of her academic program but also within the occupational therapy profession.

Empathy, professionalism, and e-professionalism

Occupational therapy straddles both the medical and social models of healthcare delivery by recognizing the importance of interpersonal skills such as empathetic interactions and therapeutic use of self to fulfill the profession's code of ethics (American Occupational Therapy Association, 2022). Indicators of such skills are described in the OT practice framework and are tracked throughout didactic education (e.g. assignments within the curriculum) and performance indicators within fieldwork education (fieldwork evaluation forms). These indicators are meant to measure students' professional skills when interacting with classmates, co-workers, instructors, clients, and other healthcare professionals (i.e. professionalism) and when interacting with others over digital platforms such as online messaging and communication, documentation, tele-learning, telehealth, and digital social interaction (i.e. e-professionalism).

Empathy extends beyond the physical context of interpersonal interaction and includes the digital context of communication, such as online learning/co-learning, social media, and telehealth practices (i.e. e-professionalism). This is important given the increasing demand for digital platforms for learning in higher education and clinical practice. E-professionalism is the display of professional paradigms that are translated into digital contexts (Alber *et al.*, 2015). Nowadays, it is hard to imagine learning without digital platforms (often referred to as Web 2.0 technologies) such as search engines, writing software, clinical simulations, and audio-visual multimedia. The integration of digital technologies within health science education has also transformed how professionalism and related competencies are embodied and developed, referred to as digital citizenship (Zhu *et al.*, 2020).

Empathy and accountability, and digital citizenship

Social media competency refers to an individual's ability to effectively and responsibly use social media platforms for various purposes, such as communication, networking, information dissemination, and professional development. It involves understanding the features and functionalities of different social media platforms, knowing how to navigate privacy settings, and utilizing appropriate etiquette and behavior online.

In a professional context, social media competency includes the following skills (Alber *et al.*, 2015):

- **Content creation:** Creating engaging and relevant content tailored to the target audience on social media platforms.

- **Audience engagement:** Interacting with followers, responding to comments and messages, and fostering meaningful conversations.

- **Brand management:** Managing the online presence and reputation of oneself or an organization, ensuring consistency and authenticity across different social media channels.

- **Analytics and insights:** Analyzing metrics and data to track the performance of social media efforts and make informed decisions for improvement.

- **Ethical considerations:** Understanding and adhering to ethical guidelines and professional standards when using social media, including patient confidentiality and privacy concerns in healthcare settings.

- **Crisis management:** Being prepared to handle and mitigate any negative feedback or crises that may arise on social media platforms.

- **Continuous learning:** Keeping up-to-date with emerging trends, features, and best practices in social media marketing and communication.

An occupational therapy student can increase their social media competency through the following steps (Kaur *et al.*, 2018):

- **Educate yourself:** Familiarize yourself with different social media platforms, their features, and their uses in healthcare and professional settings.

- **Follow relevant accounts:** Follow reputable healthcare organizations, professionals, and academic institutions on social media platforms to stay updated on industry news, trends, and best practices.

- **Engage actively:** Engage in discussions, share insights, and participate in relevant conversations within your field of interest on social media platforms. This helps you build connections and establish yourself as a knowledgeable and engaged professional.

- **Create professional profiles:** Create and maintain professional profiles on platforms like LinkedIn, where you can showcase your skills, experiences, and achievements to potential employers or collaborators.

- **Curate content:** Share relevant articles, research findings, and resources related to healthcare topics you are passionate about. Curating content demonstrates your knowledge and expertise in your field.

- **Practice ethical behavior:** Adhere to ethical guidelines and professional standards when using social media, especially about patient confidentiality and privacy. Avoid sharing sensitive information or engaging in unprofessional behavior online.

- **Attend workshops and webinars:** Take advantage of workshops, webinars, and online courses that focus on social media competency for healthcare professionals. These resources can provide valuable insights and practical tips for leveraging social media effectively in your career.

- **Network strategically:** Use social media platforms to network with peers, mentors, and professionals in your field. Building a strong professional network can open up opportunities for collaboration, mentorship, and career advancement.

- **Stay updated:** Stay informed about emerging trends, tools, and best practices in social media marketing and communication. Follow industry publications, attend conferences, and participate in online forums to stay updated on the latest developments.

- **Seek feedback:** Solicit feedback from peers, mentors, or professionals in your network to improve your social media presence and communication skills. Constructive feedback can help you identify areas for growth and refinement.

In conjunction with the use of social media technologies, the occupational therapy student also has digital citizenship. It encompasses various aspects of online behavior, including how individuals interact with others, consume and share information, and navigate digital spaces. Here are some key elements of digital citizenship (Xu *et al.*, 2019):

- **Digital literacy:** Understanding how to effectively use digital tools, navigate online platforms, and critically evaluate digital content for accuracy and reliability.

- **Responsible online behavior:** Practicing respectful and ethical conduct in online interactions, such as being mindful of others' privacy, refraining from cyberbullying, and avoiding the spread of misinformation or hate speech.

- **Protecting personal information:** Safeguarding personal data and privacy online by using strong passwords, being cautious about sharing sensitive information, and understanding privacy settings on digital platforms.

- **Cybersecurity awareness:** Being aware of potential online threats, such as phishing scams, malware, and identity theft, and taking proactive measures to protect against them, such as installing anti-virus software and keeping software up to date.

- **Digital footprint management:** Understanding that online actions leave a digital footprint and being mindful of the long-term impact of one's digital presence, including how it may affect future opportunities and relationships.

- **Respecting copyright and intellectual property:** Respecting the intellectual property rights of others by obtaining permission before using or sharing copyrighted materials online and giving proper attribution when necessary.

- **Critical thinking and media literacy:** Developing the ability to critically evaluate information and media encountered online, discerning between fact and opinion, and being skeptical of sources that lack credibility or bias.

- **Promoting digital inclusion:** Advocating for equal access to technology and digital resources for all individuals, regardless of socioeconomic status, geographic location, or other barriers.

- **Participation and collaboration:** Engaging in online communities and digital platforms constructively and collaboratively, contributing positively to discussions, and respecting diverse viewpoints.

- **Continuous learning and adaptation:** Recognizing that technology and digital landscapes are constantly evolving, and committing to ongoing learning and adaptation to stay informed and adept in digital environments.

Reflect on these questions

- Do you use social media technologies as an occupational therapy student? Why or why not?
- Is there a technological literacy for using these technologies?
- Could social media technology bridge the gap within any areas of occupational therapy education or research?

Table 3.6 outlines four core characteristics of social media competency as defined by Zhu *et al.* (2020): technical usability, content interpretation, content generation, and anticipatory reflection. Each characteristic is paired with reflective considerations to prompt critical thinking, such as the need for digital literacy and awareness of online perceptions. These components emphasize that effective engagement with social media requires not only technical skills but also thoughtful judgment and ethical reflection, especially relevant for college students preparing for professional roles.

Table 6.2: Social Media Competency Scale,
College Students (Zhu *et al.*, 2020)

Characteristics	Definitions (Zhu *et al.*, 2020)	Reflective considerations
Technical usability	The ability to operate in social media environments.	Is there a learning curve for the use of social media technologies? Should one have digital literacy?
Content interpretation	The ability to filter through content and extract appropriate meanings.	How do you validate online information to be reliable for any part of the occupational therapy process?
Content generation	The ability to communicate, convey beliefs and meaningfully negotiate with others.	Does the skill change based on the social media platform?
Anticipatory reflection	The ability to be self-aware of one's actions and others' perceptions before generating social media content.	Why should you reflect?

CASE EXAMPLE 6.2: Jennie, Malik, and Christopher are not getting along

Malik and Christopher are connected with Jennie on various social media platforms and notice her comment about one of their professors. They know Jennie has a public profile on this particular social media platform and she has also listed which academic program she is attending. Malik and Christopher are upset that Jennie is taking her issues to the online context and are concerned that their faculty member and program are being targeted. They attempt to talk to Jennie but she is very dismissive. Christopher considers taking this to the chair of the program and Malik is also convinced that this is the correct course of action.

Reflective pause

- Is Jennie within her rights to express herself on social media?
- Will Christopher and Malik be targeted for their actions if they go to the program chair?
- Which occupational therapy code of ethics is Jennie potentially violating in this situation?

Commentary on Case example 6.2

The concept of freedom of speech is a highly debated and controversial topic that requires a deeper understanding of the fundamentals of human rights, constitutional privileges, rights, and accountabilities as well as civic behavior and morals. Expressing oneself is indeed inherently supported; in fact, in occupational therapy, self-advocacy and advocating for those you serve are a distinct characteristic of the profession. However, the digital context can often blur the lines for many who wish to express themselves and believe they are excluded from the penalties attached to defamation, slander, negligence, and violations of ethics and professional conduct for healthcare practitioners. In this situation, Jennie has every right to express herself within the digital context in accordance with the rules, regulations, and policies of that social media platform; however, through publicizing her affiliation to her academic program, her remarks and statements, albeit within her rights, could be perceived as targeted harassment and in violation of any professional codes of conduct set forth by her institution. Instead, Jennie should seek to have an active dialogue with her professor and even request a moderator if need be to help facilitate the conversation productively. Embracing questions and having an open and active dialogue within a safe space is also an opportunity for Jennie to practice those critical interpersonal skills that are often utilized within the therapeutic process.

Let's think about it

Jennie and Elizabeth find themselves in a personal conflict that is tied into a professional, moral, and ethical dilemma. Should they embrace their autonomy of freedom of expression and utilize social media platforms without a correlation to their roles as occupational therapy students? Or should they start to employ conflict resolution skills, use empathy and reflection, and begin to embrace a reflective state of clinical empathy (as occupational therapy students) to better understand Dr. Taylor's actions and act accordingly? The profession's code of ethics is applicable within academic, clinical, and non-clinical spaces. This is the blueprint that guides both professional and ethical behavior among students and practitioners and if we extend our actions from the physical context to the digital, then the replication and accountability of our actions must be the same.

Recap

This scenario describes a critical time in the instances of how empathy, sympathy, and professionalism can impact the decision-making capacities of the occupational therapy student within both academic and non-academic spaces.

Reflective thinking

- Do you believe Jennie violates any code of ethics when conveying that message about a faculty member on a public social media site?

Critical thinking

- Identify an appropriate course of action Jennie and Elizabeth could take when arriving late to class and what its relevance is (if any) to clinical education.

Action-oriented thinking

- Think of one action Elizabeth can take in the *classroom* to address this experience (e.g. address this issue in a classroom conversation).
- Think of one action Jennie can take at the program level to address this experience (e.g. talk to Dr. Taylor).

HOT TAKE

Can you show clinical empathy toward someone whose identity challenges your core values?

Suggested reading to navigate this question: "Your pain is not mine: A critique of clinical empathy" (Stefanello, 2022).

References

Alber, J. M., Bernhardt, J. M., Stellefson, M., Weiler, R. M., *et al.* (2015). Designing and testing an inventory for measuring the social media competency of certified health education specialists. *Journal of Medical Internet Research*, 17(9), e221. doi: 10.2196/jmir.4943

American Occupational Therapy Association. (2020). *Occupational Therapy Code of Ethics*. *American Journal of Occupational Therapy, 74*(Supplement_3), 7413410005p1-7413410005p13. https://doi.org/10.5014/ajot.2020.74S3006

Aring, C. D. (1958). Sympathy and empathy. *Journal of the American Medical Association, 167*(4), 448-452. doi: 10.1001/jama.1958.02990210034008

Berger, D. M. (1987). *Clinical Empathy*. Jason Aronson.

Boyleo, E. J., Ting, L., & Wade, K. (2018). Predicting empathy in helping professionals: Comparison of social work and nursing students. *Social Work Education, 37*(2), 173-189. https://doi.org/10.1080/02615479.2017.1389879

Hojat, M., DeSantis, J., Shannon, S., Mortensen, L. H., *et al.* (2018). The Jefferson Scale of Empathy: A nationwide study of measurement properties, underlying components, latent variable structure, and national norm in medical students. *Advances in Health Sciences Education Theory & Practice, 23*, 899-920. https://doi.org/10.1007/s10459-018-9839-9

Hojat, M., Shannon, S. C., DeSantis, J., Shannon, S., *et al.* (2020). Empathy as related to gender, age, race and ethnicity, academic background, and career interest: A nationwide study of osteopathic medical students in the United States. *Medical Education, 54*, 571-581. https://doi.org/10.1111/medu.14138

Irving, P. & Dickson, D. (2004). Empathy: Towards a conceptual framework for health professionals. *International Journal of Health Care Quality Assurance, 17*(4-5), 212-220. doi: 10.1108/09526860410541531

Kaur, I., Shri, C., & Mital, K. M. (2018). Performance management model for teachers based on emotional intelligence and social media competencies. *Journal of Advances in Management Research, 15*(4), 414-433. https://doi.org/10.1108/JAMR-09-2017-0086

King, S. & Holosko, M. J. (2011). The development and initial validation of the empathy scale for social workers. *Research on Social Work Practice, 22*(2), 174-185. doi: 10.1177/1049731511417136

MacFarlane, P., Anderson, T., & McClintock, A. S. (2017). Empathy from the client's perspective: A grounded theory analysis. *Psychotherapy Research, 27*(2), 227-238. doi: 10.1080/10503307.2015.1090038

McNulty, J. P. & Politis, Y. (2023). Empathy, emotional intelligence, and interprofessional skills in healthcare education. *Journal of Medical Imaging and Radiation Sciences, 54*(2), 238-246. https://doi.org/10.1016/j.jmir.2023.02.014

Rogers, C. R. (1975). Empathic: An unappreciated way of being. *The Counseling Psychologist, 5*(2), 2-10. https://doi.org/10.1177/001100007500500202

Samarasekera, D. D., Lee, S. S., Yeo, J. H. T., Yeo, S. P., & Ponnamperuma, G. (2023). Empathy in health professions education: What works, gaps and areas for improvement. *Medical Education, 57*(1), 86-101. https://doi.org/10.1111/medu.14865

Stanley, S., Mettilda Buvaneswari, G., & Meenakshi, A. (2020). Predictors of empathy in women social workers. *Journal of Social Work, 20*(1), 43-63. https://doi.org/10.1177/1468017318794280

Steffanello, E. (2022). Your pain is not mine: A critique of clinical empathy. *Bioethics, 36*(5), 486-493. doi: 10.1111/bioe.12980.

Tan, L., Le, M. K., Yu, C. C., Liaw, S. Y., *et al.* (2021). Defining clinical empathy: A grounded theory approach from the perspective of healthcare workers and patients in a multicultural setting. *BMJ Open, 11*(9), e045224. https://doi.org/10.1136/bmjopen-2020-045224

Xu, S., Yang, H. H., MacLeod, J., & Zhu, S. (2019). Social media competence and digital citizenship among college students. *Convergence, 25*(4), 735-752. https://doi.org/10.1177/1354856517751390

Winter, R., Issa, E., Roberts, N., Norman, R. I., & Howick, J. (2020). Assessing the effect of empathy-enhancing interventions in health education and training: A systematic review of randomized controlled trials. *BMJ Open, 10*(9), e036471. doi: 10.1136/bmjopen-2019-036471

Zhu, S., Hao Yang, H., Xu, S., & MacLeod, J. (2020). Understanding social media competence in higher education: Development and validation of an instrument. *Journal of Educational Computing Research, 57*(8), 1935-1955. https://doi.org/10.1177/0735633118820631

CHAPTER 7

Fieldwork and Capstone

"IT'S FIELDWORK, DON'T MAKE A FUSS"

André Johnson MS, COTA/L, ROH

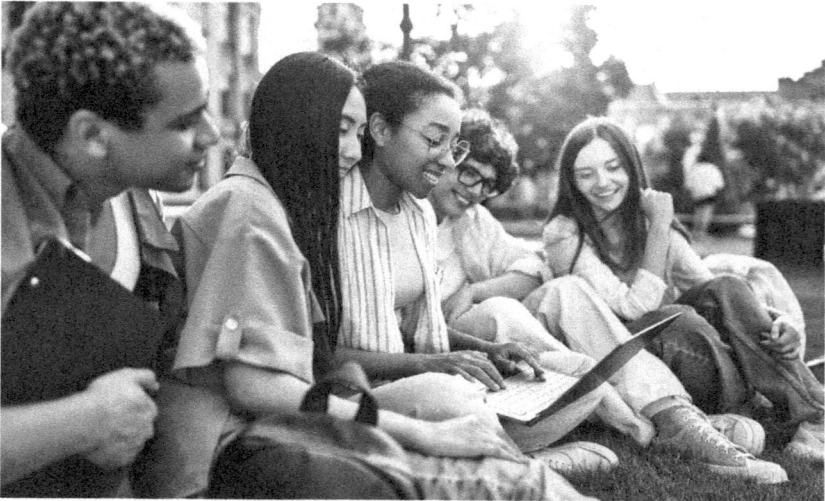

Chapter overview

This chapter connects the principles of DEI+, allyship, privilege, empathy, bias, and cultural humility in the final fieldwork component of the student academic journey within OT education. Examples of toxic and problematic interactions in fieldwork education and the capstone requirements are explored through a case-based lens. The chapter discusses strategies to identify instances lacking components of DEI+ and the concepts above to support, equip, and help students complete their fieldwork and capstone experiences as rising practitioners. Students are invited to reflect on their various levels of fieldwork experiences and capstone components.

Content

- Why fieldwork and capstones are most challenging for students.
- DEI+ in fieldwork, Case example 7.1: "You barely have an accent"
- Difficult conversations in fieldwork, Case example 7.2. "My capstone mentor called me the wrong name for a year."
- Fieldwork coordinators and educators, Case example 7.3: Allie and Dr. Boyle talk to Israa.
- De-escalation, conflict resolution, and fieldwork tips.
- Let's think about it.

Objectives

1. Identify components of DEI+ in fieldwork or capstone experiences.
2. Describe productive DEI-oriented professional behaviors in fieldwork and capstone experiences.
3. Apply strategies to address bias and discriminatory learning environments in fieldwork and capstone experiences.

Storyline snapshot

Fieldwork is a time when students put the theories and principles they have learned in their OT and OTA program into practice. DEI+ considerations do not stop once leaving the academic program. In fact, DEI+ issues are probably more prevalent and difficult to handle due to new evaluators of the student's skills in fieldwork education, and a new environment and organizational system. In this chapter, we discuss DEI+ issues through the fieldwork lens. You will be reacquainted with Cheyenne, who identifies as Indigenous, and Israa, who identifies as White North African and Muslim; their stories will guide us through everyday fieldwork experiences traversing DEI+ issues.

Characters in this chapter (see character matrix in Appendix 2 for details)

- Allie

- Gemma
- Lauren
- Cheyenne
- Israa
- Lin
- Dr. Boyle
- Dr. Joseph
- Dr. Klein

Fieldwork: The journey, experience, and entry into the profession

Education is for improving the lives of others and for leaving your community and world better than you found it.

MARIAN WRIGHT EDELMAN

The voyage through occupational therapy education and its impact on the student's eventual frontline clinician professional career starts within occupational therapy programmatic/didactic learning. Most experiences in which students truly learn and grow in academic environments have been thought through, carefully planned, tried, and tested by educational programs. The outcomes of these experiences are not by happenstance. The experiences students encounter have been formulated for success "within a controlled environment" in most occupational therapy OT and OTA academic programs. Meanwhile, students' fieldwork and capstone experience placements are in real-life environments, where different variables come into play, and quick, effective decision-making is critical.

While issues related to DEI+ are key aspects in healthcare, and the majority of workers (56%) believe that an increased focus on DEI+ is a good direction, 44% think that it has a neutral effect or consider it "bad," demonstrating that the subject remains highly polarizing (Minkin, 2023).

Further evidence illustrating the polarization of DEI+ is an American Hospital Association report (2024), which found that only 55% of hospital healthcare systems had a DEI+ strategic plan to address diversity from historically marginalized populations. This results in a unique dynamic environment where a student must apply the foundational principles they have learned for success in the academic environment while having to navigate DEI+ issues. Students must now translate and generalize learned skills while utilizing ethical decision-making in a real-world environment not as attuned to their cultural and specific needs. This can be particularly challenging given the intricate nature of DEI+ issues and the role of culture in daily functioning within clinical practice.

Academic fieldwork coordinators

Academic fieldwork coordinators (AFWCs) are mandatory full-time positions in any occupational therapy educational program, and the role is a highly dynamic and constantly changing one. It is also a role in which the complete set of duties and responsibilities is not fully understood by other faculty members or even, at times, the program director. AFWCs must understand academic institutional standards and the many different clinical site requirements, processes, and timeframes involved. They must market and advocate for the program and work collaboratively to acquire affiliation agreements; they must obtain Level I and Level II placements that, many times, must be requested in a systematic way a year or two or more in advance, particularly if the sites to be acquired are in high demand and are desired Level I or Level II placements.

Additionally, AFWCs must strongly consider an organization's mission and value, combined with the academic institution's mission and value, and match that to a student's setting preferences, early career ambitions, and overall unique portfolio of talents, characteristics, skills, needs, and accommodations. Accommodations, for example, while legally and on the surface are understood and ensured to be followed in practice, do not always equivocally translate to real-world demands. Additionally, accommodations require sustained efforts by the student and AFWC to be addressed and implemented correctly. AFWCs must foster a relationship with a student when, at times, they have the least physical time with said student compared to other faculty previously encountered during earlier didactic learning. This lack of being seen is not due to a lack of work at hand. They also navigate the meeting of academic institution requirements, attend mandatory meetings, teach workloads, and make phone calls and send emails while keeping an eye on all students who are out in clinical fieldwork. Part of the AFWC's role is to ensure that support, encouragement, critical feedback, and success strategies are available to students and fieldwork educators when needed.

Additionally, the AFWC must provide a spectrum of fieldwork opportunities representing the clients, communities, and populations being served locally and regionally, as well as fieldwork opportunities that facilitate success for all program students (Nuwere *et al.*, 2022). Considerations must be made reasonably for cultural, spiritual, and personal needs. For example, are all clinical sites accessible? Are unseen disabilities considered and understood at all facilities? How will a student's academic accommodations mesh with the clinical environment? Will they be adhered to? These questions are critically important for the AFWC to address to ensure the student's optimal transition to the clinical environment for Level I and II fieldwork experiences. Table 7.1 describes terms related to different roles in fieldwork education.

Fieldwork educators and capstone educators

Fieldwork educators (FWEs) and capstone educators are critical to student development. They authentically must strive for student success with a genuine commitment to the student's professional development. FWEs must do all this while creating a learning environment and, at times, navigating a very stressful clinical environment where productivity, staffing demands, or administration or institutional pressures are occurring. The AFWC role is a challenging one that comes with a lot of power, and all parties involved must consider these effects. The student and the fieldwork educator will form a relationship that will indelibly impact the beginning of the student's career. Consider for a moment that this is perhaps the student's first full-time exposure to the profession and that the individuals shaping their future have very little information about this person they might have just met, except for exposure to the person when reviewing the initial fieldwork objectives' sign-off. FWEs have great power in this setup and vouch for their professional support of the student to capably enter the profession in specific timeframes, ranging from 8 weeks for OTAs, to 12 weeks for OTs, or 14 weeks for the capstone experience (American Occupational Therapy Association, 2023a, 2023b). The FWE must be aware of the power dynamic and the environment of the fieldwork student. It is something that all parties involved should discuss for clarity of expectations. Consideration should be given to issues such as when feedback will be provided, and if it will be in front of a client or not. Perhaps this is only done when a situation involving safety or a similar level of concern necessitates it. Also, what is the student's optimal learning style for growth and success? Discussions about "professionalism" and expectations should be fully acknowledged between the student and FWE before day 1 when site-specific objectives are signed.

Doctoral capstone coordinator

Doctoral capstone coordinator (DCC) is a mandatory full-time position in any occupational therapy doctorate program. The doctoral capstone coordinator is not to be confused with the academic fieldwork coordinator position as their position is different, involving different priorities and objectives for the student. The DCC is one of the leadership positions in the department and maintains the responsibility to create, implement, and oversee all capstone experiences according to ACOTE standard A.2.5. (American Occupational Therapy Association, 2023b). The DCC position is skilled at programmatic evaluation and determining outcomes in collaboration with the program director and the academic fieldwork coordinator in accordance with ACOTE standards (Accreditation Council for Occupational Therapy Education, 2018). The 14-week capstone experience, unlike fieldwork experiences, is collaboratively designed and individualized to the student for this learning opportunity. These capstone experiences enable students to design and implement innovative, student-led solutions within emerging areas of occupational therapy practice. The professional relationship between the DCC capstone coordinator, the capstone mentor, and the student must be fostered like that of the academic fieldwork coordinator.

Lastly, and most importantly, we have the students in the fieldwork and capstone process. The fieldwork experience has an exciting and challenging dynamic. Students must navigate a professionally challenging yet career-altering relationship that offers essential fundamental lessons; at the same time, the person mentoring the student's experience is a new individual they are getting used to. The student is also potentially acclimatizing to a new area where they undertake their fieldwork experience with inconsistent social support and limited resources. It is critical to have open and transparent conversations and written expectations regarding Level I and Level II placements and where they will be held. Consider that the student may be entering a full-time healthcare setting for the first time, adapting to a new geographic location, working under the evaluation of an unfamiliar supervisor, and facing high stakes that could determine their ability to progress toward their chosen career. Additionally, the financial constraint of this opportunity is a barrier and should be a consideration for every student.

Conversely, it is essential that students demonstrate intentionality in their desire to learn from the fieldwork or capstone educator, as this directly supports their ability to optimize care for the clients they will eventually treat and serve. Effectively explaining why an action was performed is critical to the occupational therapy fieldwork experience. Students must also be prepared for core foundational elements of the profession to be learned during their fieldwork placements or capstone experiences. The core elements should be covered during previous didactic classes within the curriculum. Many aspects of the fieldwork experience will need to be learned on the fieldwork experience. Still, foundational underpinnings of the profession and settings in which the student is placed need to be adequately reviewed and covered to set the student up for optimal learning and occupational performance in the fieldwork or capstone environment.

Personal biases, expectations, and disabilities, seen and unseen, must be considered by all parties in the fieldwork and capstone process. Clear, objective communication is critical in fostering the therapeutic relationship between the student and all parties.

Table 7.1: Terms and roles related to fieldwork education in occupational therapy

Term	Description	Roles and responsibilities
Academic fieldwork coordinator (AFWC)	This individual or team of individuals in OT and OTA programs is necessary and mandatory in occupational therapy academic education. Primary responsibilities are adherence to all C standards from the Accreditation Council of Occupational Therapy Education (American Occupational Therapy Association, 2023a).	The AFWC directly addresses fieldwork education, student support, marketing, contracts, partnerships, advocacy, and student fieldwork placements for the OT/OTA academic programs. They are the critical primary contact, support, and ally for all DEI+ issues occurring on Level I and II fieldwork.
Doctoral capstone coordinator (DCC)	This individual or team of individuals in occupational therapist and occupational therapy assistant programs is another necessary and mandatory position within occupational therapy doctoral programs per the Accreditation Council of Occupational Therapy Education (ACOTE). The capstone coordinator is responsible for the ACOTE D standards. (American Occupational Therapy Association, 2023b).	The DCC possesses expertise in teaching and curricular design and redesign, capstone procedure development, and implementation of student advisement. The DCC additionally coordinates all faculty advisors and administration of the capstone experience for all eligible students. This is a critical primary contact, support, and ally for all DEI+ issues during the DCC capstone experience.

Experiential learning	The process of learning by doing. It is the hands-on experiences in real-world situations that students can reflect on to further their overall set of skills. Experiential learning occurs at times during the didactic curriculum but occurs most frequently in the clinical field.	Occupational therapy students have experiential learning opportunities in Level I and II fieldwork experience. Experiential learning is the cumulation of observation experiences and apprenticeship experiences. Level I and Level II fieldwork experiences are where most experiential learning will happen for the OT and OTA student.
Fieldwork educator (FWE)	A subject matter expert who serves as a guide, mentor, and role model for the occupational therapy student. In Level I occupational therapy experiences, this individual does not have to be an occupational therapy practitioner. In Level II occupational therapy experiences, this individual must be a licensed occupational therapist or occupational therapy assistant, depending on the educational degree being acquired.	This individual is responsible for Level I and Level II fieldwork in guiding and supporting the student during the clinical experience for optimal success in the respective setting. From a DEI+ lens, this individual wields an incredible amount of power (due to the apprenticeship model structure of fieldwork) and responsibility in the student–FWE relationship in transforming a student with practitioner foundational knowledge into an occupational therapy practitioner (OT and OTA) with entry-level skills. FWEs are usually a student's first full-time look at the current occupational practice environment, frontline practitioner morale, and the expectations of an occupational therapy practitioner.
Fieldwork performance evaluation (FWPE)	Fieldwork Performance Evaluation, the AOTA fieldwork performance evaluation tool, is utilized as an assessment to allow both the student and fieldwork educator a standardized measure for evaluating student performance in occupational therapy clinical settings or emergent practice areas.	OT and OTA students must obtain a passing score to complete their respective Level I and Level II clinical fieldwork experiences.
Student Evaluation of the Fieldwork Experience (SEFWE)	The SEFWE is an evaluation of the fieldwork experience shared with the academic fieldwork coordinator and future students in the OT and OTA program attending the site.	The SEFWE is utilized to obtain the OT student's authentic and objective overview of the FWE from the respective student's experience.

cont.

Term	Description	Roles and responsibilities
Level I and Level II fieldwork	Level I and II fieldwork experiences allow the OT student to observe OT practice while still in occupational therapy education coursework. These experiences are usually short term, and students have multiple opportunities and different settings.	The intention of Level I experiences is not to facilitate independent performance of OT skills, but to promote and facilitate OT skill development of learned principles from the academic (didactic) program. Level II experiences intend to encourage independent performance of OT skills to allow for a generalist occupational therapy practitioner. These experiences are typically two 12-week experiences for OT students and two 8-week experiences for OTA students.
Doctoral capstone experience (DCE)	In a doctoral capstone experience and project, students self-direct their learning. They also disseminate the project and demonstrate the synthesis of in-depth knowledge gained through the experience (Kroll *et al.*, 2022).	The DCE is a unique 14-week experience in OT doctoral programs. The doctoral capstone coordinator supports the experience, which is not to be considered fieldwork.
Hostile environment	A workplace environment that consists potentially of harassment, discrimination, unwelcome verbal or physical conduct, jokes, teasing, microaggressions, or acts or hazing relating to the affected individual.	This type of environment has a substantial opportunity to affect the OT student's work performance, mental health, and overall occupational well-being. Students must proactively communicate this hostile environment to the AFWC or DCC as soon as possible. The FWE, AFWC, and DCC should support, intervene, and take reasonable action to remediate or terminate the clinical placement.

DEI+ in fieldwork

DEI+ in the workplace is crucial for fostering a positive and productive environment where all employees feel valued and supported (Babatunde *et al.*, 2023). This also applies to fieldwork students, as a critical transition occurs in the clinical field. The OT/OTA student must understand that they are still under the university umbrella. Furthermore, they are now considered volunteers or employees of the organization where they perform their Level I or Level II placement. The responsibility to be prepared is not solely on the students; the academic fieldwork coordinator should educate students on this matter to ensure a smooth transition. Another vital piece of this equation is ensuring collaboration between the AFWC and students on the matching of the fieldwork site to ensure a quality fit. It is critically vital that transparent and clear expectations are understood so that students are actively prepared for the geographical area, FWE expectations, and expected behaviors at the clinical site to form an educated agreement on the fieldwork placement (Babatunde *et al.*, 2023).

Another key issue in fieldwork is the power dynamic between the FWE and student. During the fieldwork experience Level I and Level II, as in the classroom, students face a power dynamic that puts them in a subservient position, which often saps empowerment.

Hierarchical power dynamics inhibit team communication, initiation, and assertive behaviors, which impacts overall team effectiveness and patient safety. A chain is only as strong as its weakest link. This can lead to a student having feelings of intimidation and powerlessness, fears of reprisal and repercussions, perceived poor self-efficacy, and a lack of confidence and role clarity (Kearns *et al.*, 2021). This is a consideration that must be provided with didactic attention and education to facilitate the student's transition to the clinical environment.

CASE EXAMPLE 7.1: "You barely have an accent"

Gemma and her fieldwork educator, Lauren, see a patient (client) who is a native Spanish speaker and speaks very little English. The patient is learning to comply with and follow her rotator cuff repair precautions. Gemma springs into action, translating and facilitating the overall treatment session and educating the patient on her existing precautions. The following debrief conversation and feedback occur shortly after the termination of the treatment session. Lauren, the FWE, says to Gemma, "Awesome job, Gemma! Loved you stepping up and translating during the session. How did you learn to speak Spanish?" Gemma hesitates, then tactfully and professionally states, "I mentioned when I introduced myself that I was Afro-Latina and was originally born in Cuba." Lauren replies, "That's right! I just have a hard time remembering, as you barely have an accent. You're going to be a great asset to the team."

Reflective pause

- How would you describe FWE Lauren's feedback regarding Gemma's performance as an occupational therapist?
- Does the FWE provide Gemma with objective feedback?
- What do you think about Gemma? Does she handle the situation well? How might you handle this situation differently?

Commentary on Case example 7.1

This scenario describes a situation that can unfortunately occur during fieldwork experiences. The FWE does not give the student feedback on her objective core skills. Additionally, the FWE makes a comment regarding how unnoticeable Gemma's accent is, which is inappropriate as she brings more than just her language skills. That said, Gemma's handling of the situation in a professional setting is to be commended. She follows the profession's ethical principle of prudence in this scenario.

Navigating tough FW situations and de-escalation on fieldwork

Fieldwork will have many great moments, but there will perhaps be some not-so-great moments as well. How you handle these moments will, at times, have a significant impact on your journey to becoming a practitioner. Consider a situation outside the fieldwork or capstone experience in which perhaps you have received what you consider "attitude" or perhaps "a little extra" critical feedback.

Now consider the environment: hospital setting, mental health facility, community health setting, women's health clinic, outpatient clinic, school, long-term care facility, or emerging practice area. It is important to remember in all these environments that we try to handle things gracefully and consider the best intentions in situations (minus those in which personal harm is involved). Remember the health of the clients we serve and that environments are critically important to keep positive and to maintain low stress for the promotion of optimal recovery and wellness. The student's concerns are extremely important to consider as well, but it is pivotal to discuss objective information from all perspectives. Within healthcare, conflict de-escalation builds on conflict management principles, and is specifically aimed at preventing the escalation of agitation and aggression to physical violence (Rosenman *et al.*, 2017).

As occupational therapy practitioners, we are great solution finders, and finding a resolution or optimal agreement to move forward in difficult situations should be the goal if reasonably possible (Suarez-Balcazar *et al.*, 2023). Addressing conflict when it presents itself intentionally, and with the appropriate immediacy and action, is essential to addressing conflicts, particularly those involving inclusion, equity, and diversity issues with students (McArthur & Gill, 2021). Acknowledgment and addressing the problems appropriately when they do present themselves is critical for students to feel valued and respected in the clinical workplace (Babatunde *et al.*, 2023). A comprehensive debrief of the situation should be held with the AFWC to determine a collaborative plan of action and future additional steps (Marsico *et al.*, 2023). Support and clear, objective expectations should be provided for the student as needed and whenever possible.

> **CASE EXAMPLE 7.2: "My capstone mentor called me the wrong name for a year"**
> DCC capstone mentor Dr. Joseph states, "It has been great mentoring you over these last 11 months, Chuh-nai." Dr. Klein, the AFWC, who is sitting in on this particular meeting, interjects and says, "Cary, I believe it is 'Cheyenne'." Cary redirects to Cheyenne, and says, "Is it?" Cheyenne softly responds, "Yes, that is how you pronounce it." Dr. Joseph replies, "I am sorry. I cannot believe I've been saying your name incorrectly for all this time." Cheyenne replies, "It's okay."

Reflective pause

- How do you think this could have happened if this situation had played out after the FWE and the students had known each other for almost a year?
- What factors do you think led to this outcome? Have you advocated for yourself as a student in a similar situation? If so, how?
- Have you experienced a similar situation in which you might not have felt comfortable due to respect for a superior or culture, or due to a professional title?

Commentary on Case example 7.2

This scenario describes a typical situation where a name is mispronounced. The particular issue in this scenario is that the capstone mentor genuinely does not know how to pronounce Cheyenne's name. Cheyenne, in this scenario, faces a common situation in which a student perhaps does not feel comfortable correcting her professor and mentor. With that said, Cheyenne has every right over the time of her mentorship to kindly correct Dr. Joseph regarding her name; that Cheyenne does not, in this scenario, is due to a cultural perspective on respect for elders and authority and is a dynamic that faculty should consider. We could debate that Dr. Joseph could have asked for clarity prior, directly asking Cheyenne how to correctly say her name if in doubt or consulting with a faculty member. Still, taking it at face value, Dr. Joseph does handle this situation appropriately, though understandably it is embarrassing and hard to fathom that Dr. Joseph does not know a mentee's correct name pronunciation after nearly a year of working together.

Fieldwork coordinators and educators

In occupational therapy fieldwork, challenging situations will arise; there is no way around it. Students must be prepared; the relationship between the student, academic fieldwork and capstone coordinator is a vital piece in providing the student with a trusted confidant and advocate when navigating the new clinical environment. That said, the therapeutic relationship must be developed, fostered, and nurtured while the student is under academic instruction, or via alternate methods (online meetings, advisements, etc.) to ensure that trust is established. It is also beneficial for students on Level II placement, if away from home, to have a supplemental support system that can help address issues.

CASE EXAMPLE 7.3: Allie and Dr. Boyle talk to Israa

During a supervision visit to Allie's community capstone site, Dr. Boyle observes Allie's progress and checks in on her experience. While they are meeting, Israa, another MSOT student placed at the same facility, approaches and shares some concerns. She explains that she has faced discomfort with certain clients due to her spiritual clothing and feels unsupported by her fieldwork educator. When Israa brought up her concerns, the educator responded dismissively, saying, "I'm not sure how to support you with that. I guess we don't have control over what clients say about us, do we?"

Dr. Boyle and Allie listen attentively and reassure Israa that she belongs in the space and has done nothing wrong. They encourage her to speak directly with her fieldwork educator again and to reach out to the facility's human resources department. Both offer their support moving forward. Israa responds, "Thank you. I feel more confident addressing this now. I really appreciate you hearing me and reminding me that I do belong."

Reflective pause

- Have you experienced a situation similar to Israa? How did you feel, and what action did you take?
- What factors do you think led to this outcome? How have you advocated for yourself as a student in a similar situation?
- Have you experienced a similar situation in which you might not have felt comfortable due to respect for superiors, cultural differences, or due to a professional title?

Commentary on Case example 7.3

Unfortunately, this scenario describes a situation that occurs more often than we would like. Islamophobia and hate speech are on the uptick. The scenario depicts a situation in which the student is in a genuinely trying and difficult situation. Her fieldwork educator, who should have addressed the matter immediately and been supportive, has left Israa, her fieldwork student, unsupported in a situation she should have stepped in and addressed from inception; there is no doubt about this. That said, the scenario also shows the power of supporting an individual when something is not right. Dr. Boyle's and Allie's support empowers Israa to address a problematic situation and communicate accordingly with her fieldwork educator. Israa feels validated in how she feels and reassured that she belongs in this profession, although this unfortunate situation is occurring.

Fieldwork education and difficult conversations in the classroom

Fieldwork education is an opportunity for students to learn the nuances and specific skills required for practice. The fieldwork education experience can encompass fieldwork preparation, education on the onboarding process, roles and responsibilities, frontline clinical experiences, and administrative experiences that support the development of the occupational therapy student.

Occupational therapy fieldwork educators are people first, fostering, maintaining, and sustaining mature relationships with them is essential for facilitating optimal learning. Students should demonstrate an intentional nature, self-advocating in their learning and professional development process, and a desire to change, adapt, evolve, learn, and grow from their fieldwork experiences. Students must also understand that they represent themselves, the college or university, and are community partners. Therefore, it is vital to demonstrate clinical excellence, cultural humility, and professional ethics and behaviors in the fieldwork education process.

The AFWC and the student should foster an optimal professional relationship. The AFWC needs to make clear the objectives, discuss the student's preferences and career aspirations, and ensure an understanding of fieldwork expectations and transition to the clinical field for optimal conditions for the student's success. Fieldwork education by the AFWC should address all areas of the aspects mentioned above, but also include learning about and enacting practical support for different ways of engaging in basic activities of daily living (ADLs), practicing of modeling advocacy, and empowerment strategies that address systemic racism barriers that exist at varying levels of an organization. Additionally the AFWC also should provide this education to institutional fieldwork educators in an accessible format (Johnson *et al.*, 2022).

Remember, the fieldwork and capstone experiences are an opportunity that many individuals and organizations have to mutually agree to allow these Level I and Level fieldwork experiences. The fieldwork educator, however they are viewed, is committed to enabling students to treat and serve their clients. They also allow students to utilize the built-up therapeutic trust to perform an independent evaluation or treatment, or to co-treat. The patients a student assesses, evaluates, and treats have hugely contributed to the fieldwork and capstone experience and allowed the student the opportunity to help them in their recovery process.

Below are some of the tips for students to remember about fieldwork:

- There are always multiple perspectives to a situation. Process the actions, events, and behaviors, self-reflect objectively, and consider both sides.
- Create a professional support system consisting of occupational therapy practitioners and other external professionals to draw on during fieldwork education and in the early stages of your career.
- Keep lines of communication open at all times. Contact the AFWC, DDC, and FWE and communicate needs and concerns during fieldwork education and capstone experiences.

Let's think about it

Gemma and Lin are on Level II fieldwork at an outpatient hand facility. It is the Friday before Martin Luther King Jr. (MLK) Day weekend and the end of the first week of their Level II placement. Lin's fieldwork educator wishes Lin a wonderful holiday weekend, and Lin quickly wraps up and leaves the facility. Gemma's fieldwork educator chooses to debrief her on her performance for the week before the holiday weekend. The feedback overall is that Gemma is doing well on her Level II experience. At the end of the meeting, Gemma's fieldwork educator asks, "What are you doing for MLK Day?" Gemma responds, "I am just going to take it easy." (Gemma has service commitments for Monday but feels most comfortable disclosing that she will take it easy.) Gemma's fieldwork educator responds, "Really? It's MLK weekend; I thought it was a big day for the Black/African American community." She continues, "Martin Luther King Jr. is a significant figure. I am surprised you're not doing something else." Gemma says, "I am going to take the time for myself for my work/life balance, since I am doing fieldwork." The conversation concludes. On leaving the facility, Gemma calls Lin to brief her of the situation and informs her she did not appreciate the comments regarding her MLK weekend plans as she is Black-Latina and does not only identify with the Black/African American community. She feels that her fieldwork educator went too far and was intrusive. Lin replies, "I understand, Gemma. Perhaps you should tell Dr. Klein (AFWC) about the situation." Gemma agrees, and the conversation ends shortly afterward.

Reflective thinking

- What do you think about this interaction and Gemma's concerns?
- What steps would you take in this situation?

Critical thinking questions

- Challenging situations will occur like this via a poor relationship with your prospective fieldwork educator, difficult moments with a client, or simply a lousy personal day.
  - What de-escalation or conflict-resolution skills do you have?
- Do you have a good relationship with your AFWC? Why do you think this is important?

Action-oriented thinking

- Think of one action Gemma should take to address her concerns. Please fully explain.

HOT TAKE

Our mental health and the connection to DEI+ in the workplace.

Read: "The intersection between mental health and DEIA in the OT workplace" (Wells, 2023).

References

Accreditation Council for Occupational Therapy Education (2023). 2023 Accreditation Council for Occupational Therapy Education (ACOTE®) Standards and Interpretive Guide (effective July 31, 2025). https://acoteonline.org/accreditation-explained/standards

American Hospital Association. (2024). *Institute for Diversity and Health Equity.* https://ifdhe.aha.org

American Journal of Occupational Therapy, 78(1), 7810410100. https://doi.org/10.5014/ajot.2024.78S102

American Occupational Therapy Association. (2023a). *Overview of roles and responsibilities of the academic fieldwork coordinator.* www.aota.org/-/media/corporate/files/educationcareers/coe/coe_afwc-roles-2023-final.pdf

American Occupational Therapy Association. (2023b). *Overview of roles and responsibilities of the doctoral capstone coordinator.* www.aota.org/-/media/corporate/files/educationcareers/coe/coe_dcc-roles-2023-final.pdf

Babatunde, F., Dasola, H. A., & Adeshina, O. (2023). Managing conflicts arising from diversity and inclusion policies at workplace. *International Journal for Social Studies, 9*(3), 15–30. https://doi.org/10.5281/zenodo.7843489

Johnson, K. R., Kirby, A., Washington, S., Lavalley, R., & Faison, T. (2022). Linking antiracist action from the classroom to practice. *American Journal of Occupational Therapy, 76*(5), 7605347010. https://doi.org/10.5014/ajot.2022.050054

Kearns, E., Khurshid, Z., Anjara, S., De Brún, A., Rowan, B., & McAuliffe, E. (2021). P92 Power dynamics in healthcare teams: A barrier to team effectiveness and patient safety: A systematic review. *BJS Open, 5*(Suppl 1), zrab032.091. https://doi.org/10.1093/bjsopen/zrab032.091

Kroll, C., Struckmeyer, L. R., & Schmeltz, B. (2022). What is the entry-level OTD doctoral capstone and how can you benefit? Aota.org. www.aota.org/publications/ot-practice/ot-practice-issues/2022/entry-level-otd-capstone

Marsico, A. M., Lekovitch, C., & Raina, K. (2023). Aota.org. www.aota.org/publications/ot-practice/ot-practice-issues/2023/stop-talk-roll-a-framework-for-students-in-fieldwork

McArthur, A. R. & Gill, C. J. (2021). Building bridges: Integrating disability ethics into occupational therapy practice. *American Journal of Occupational Therapy, 75*(4), 7504347010. https://doi.org/10.5014/ajot.2021.044164

Minkin, R. (2023). *Diversity, Equity, and Inclusion in the Workplace.* PEW Research Center. www.pewresearch.org/social-trends/2023/05/17/diversity-equity-and-inclusion-in-the-workplace

Nuwere, E., Wheeler, A., & Darko, J. (2022). Pipeline to the future: Increasing fieldwork opportunities for underrepresented OT students. *OT Practice.* www.aota.org/publications/ot-practice/ot-practice-issues/2022/fieldwork-dei-initiative

Rosenman, E. D., Vrablik, M. C., Charlton, P. W., Chipman, A. K., & Fernandez, R. (2017). Promoting workplace safety: Teaching conflict management and de-escalation skills in graduate medical education. *Journal of Graduate Medical Education, 9*(5), 562–566. https://doi.org/10.4300/JGME-D-17-00006.1

Suarez-Balcazar, Y., Arias, D., & Munoz, J. (2023). Promoting justice, diversity, equity, and inclusion through caring communities: Why it matters to occupational therapy. *American Journal of Occupational Therapy, 77*(6), 7706347020. https://doi.org/10.5014/ajot.2023.050416

Wells, S. A. (2023). The intersection between mental health and DEIA in the OT workplace. *SIS Quarterly: Mental Health.* www.aota.org/publications/sis-quarterly/mental-health-sis/mhsis-2-23

CHAPTER 8

Student to Clinician

To all the Allies and Gemmas

Razan Hamed PhD., OTR/L
and Vikram Pagpatan EdD., OTR/L, FAOTA

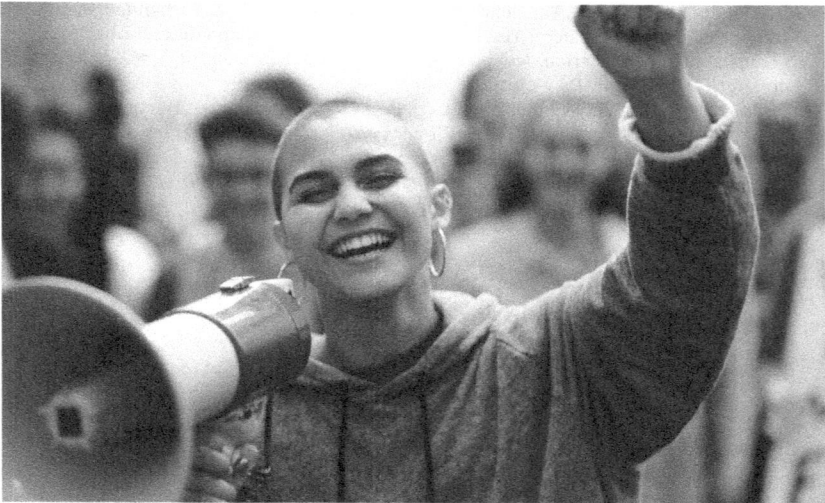

Chapter overview

This chapter walks the student through the journey of transforming into an ethical and DEI+ mindful practitioner. The chapter highlights the variations in growth among students and the need to constantly pursue opportunities for self-expansion in DEI+. Examples of professional engagement opportunities within AOTA, community groups, and state associations to instill lifelong advocacy and growth are identified. Students are invited to explore opportunities for future growth in the DEI+ arena, such as identifying mentorship, research opportunities related to social change, and professional engagement in community-centered practices.

- From the classroom to the clinic, Case example 8.1: Rehashing the OT school journey.
- Transition versus transformation.
- Professional development, engagement, and DEI+, Case example 8.2: Fares and Hana hold a multi-faith panel.
- The first-year as an occupational therapy practitioner, Case example 8.3: "Jade, you speak like a White girl!"
- DEI+, AAA, and culture change—how does the journey continue? Case example 8.4: Ashwayna runs for state board elections.
- DEI+ and the next generations of OTS, Case example 8.5: Allie and Gemma meet with the new students and share the lessons learned during their OT studies.
- Let's think about it.

Objectives

1. Identify challenging aspects of transitioning into the clinician and professional roles.
2. Describe professional development behaviors that can enhance DEI+ in the profession.
3. Apply strategies to address potential bias and discriminatory working environments.

Storyline snapshot

It is the end of the school journey for Allie and Gemma. They are not the same individuals who started the OT program two years ago. Together, they worked on assignments, laughed, cried, and complained about professors and exams. They had fun conversations and tough dialogues. Some were pleasant and others were challenging, yet all were insightful and self-expanding. Now the two embark on the next step toward becoming an OT practitioner. The goals they have in mind are similar in some ways—certification, licensure, job, family, and life. Yet how they navigate these goals is tangled with the intricate web of their intersectionalities. They both have dreams, aspirations, and plans but the worries that lie ahead for these two students in the OT world are far from similar.

To all the Allies and Gemmas out there, you are not alone...

Characters in this chapter (see character matrix in Appendix 2 for details)

- Allie
- Gemma
- Fares
- Hana
- Ashwayna (Ash)
- Dr. Campbell
- Dr. Cruz
- Jade

From the classroom to the clinic

Every great dream begins with a dreamer. Always remember, you have within you the strength, the patience, and the passion to reach for the stars to change the world.

HARRIET TUBMAN

While transitioning from the student to the practitioner role can be exciting for many students, it can be anxiety-provoking for others (Opoku *et al.*, 2021). Students' concerns may include readiness to start unsupervised clinical practice, juggling life and career goals, financial stability, and the physical and mental burden of the job (Moir *et al.*, 2021). Other concerns may include the gap between education and practice, fitting into the work culture, or managing client caseload. In some cases, the gap between the classroom and the clinical environment may include issues related to DEI+ that can make the transition even more complicated. The following are a few examples:

- Workplace policies around religious or cultural practices (e.g. granting days off and honoring non-major religious or cultural observations such as Lunar Year, Diwali, and Nowruz).

- Resources available to support aspects of DEI+ (e.g. presence of affinity group).
- Established practices supporting marginalized identities (e.g. availability of inclusive restrooms or regulatory paperwork acknowledging non-binary identities).
- State-sanctioned policies supporting marginalized communities (e.g. work policy on hiring transgender individuals).

Regardless of the gap between the classroom and the clinic, students must identify their needs and seek support while advocating for safe and inclusive work environments that are conducive to productive clinical practice.

CASE EXAMPLE 8.1: Rehashing the OT school journey

It is the last day of fieldwork Level II for Allie and Gemma. They are meeting with their academic advisor to rehash their experience and get ready for the next steps toward board examination and licensure. During the meeting with her advisor Allie shares that she is excited for the next chapter in her OT journey, albeit slightly anxious about taking the board exam. She describes her timeline for taking the exam and some study tools she found on the AOTA and the National Board for Certification in Occupational Therapy (NBCOT) websites. Gemma meets with her advisor and shares similar plans to Allie's but she also goes on to talk about anxiety, finding support similar to what she has had during OT school. She states, "Not that school was perfect, to be honest, but I mean at least there is COTAD [the Coalition of Occupational Therapy Advocates for Diversity], you [the advisor], the affinity groups, and overall a sense of a guarded learning space. I am not sure what I will be dealing with when I land my first job."

Reflective pause

- How are Allie's and Gemma's concerns similar and different?
- Which one of these concerns is similar to or different from your concerns, or a current student's?
- What advice would you give both students while they prepare for the next chapter of their OT career?

Commentary on Case example 8.1

The scenario describes an example of the type of concerns students share when they transition to the clinic. While the students share similar concerns to an extent, Gemma has an additional concern about socio-emotional support. No longer being part of a group or experiencing the protected classroom atmosphere and supportive spaces are common concerns shared by students of marginalized communities. New clinicians who share similar concerns to Gemma's can identify a goal of seeking or identifying similar support spaces or groups. Seeking mentorship, trusted allies, or friends could be a good goal for the first year of clinical practice. Establishing a professional support space can enhance their sense of confidence and belonging and may boost their potential as social agents of change who serve DEI+ issues (Picotin *et al.*, 2021).

Transition versus transformation

Occupational therapy practitioners work with individuals of different backgrounds, including age, gender, race, faith, ability, and other aspects of diversity. Hence, being a DEI+ mindful practitioner involves an ethical obligation to uphold the core values and principles constituting the profession's code of ethics. Being DEI+ mindful is a journey and a mindset that does not readily happen when students transition into the clinician role. It is an approach to practice that necessitates self-awareness of bias and professional strengths and limitations. For example, failure to recognize one's biases or lack of experience in a practice area may affect service provision (e.g. violating nonmaleficence in the code of ethics).

Being DEI+ mindful also requires awareness of events affecting healthcare (including OT practices) such as local, national, and global movements, legislations, and laws. Oblivion to these events may blindside the practitioner on matters affecting clients' daily lives and thus their functioning and access to OT services. Eventually, this may undermine the ethical principles of the OT profession. For example, ignoring legislation governing health or insurance coverage for undocumented immigrants or refugees may limit the occupational therapy practitioner's ability to uphold the ethical principle of justice in the profession's code of ethics (i.e. promoting equity, inclusion, and unbiased provision of care).

Most educational programs intentionally prepare students for transitioning into the clinician role by addressing issues related to board examinations, licensure, job interviews, resume writing, and professional development. However, rarely are students prepared for the *practitioner* role, which calls for a professional transformation rather than merely transitioning to "clinical personnel." Transforming into a professional means proactively considering issues beyond daily clinical practice such as DEI+ issues, growth mindset, leadership, advocacy, and social justice. Although lightly discussed in most OT curricula, these issues are beyond the educational and clinical content required by accrediting bodies in occupational therapy (e.g. the Accreditation Council of Occupational Therapy Education) or those in higher education (e.g. the Department of Higher Education). Therefore, students tend to pay less attention to DEI+ mindful practices such as cultural humility, allyship, and professional engagement once they enter clinical practice. The difference between transitioning into a clinician and transforming into a practitioner requires the active ongoing learning of issues related not only to daily practice but also to issues affecting their clients that may not be visible to the naked eye (e.g. limited access to health literacy due to their citizenship status).

The larger picture

Being a DEI+ mindful occupational therapy practitioner makes the OT community better connected as we learn from one another. Practitioners can promote DEI+ mindful practices within their practice areas, sharing knowledge with peers, clients, and other stakeholders on issues related to DEI+. The following are some examples of practical steps new practitioners can take to support their (and others') transformation toward DEI+ in clinical practice:

- Providing in-service training to colleagues and staff on practical issues related to DEI+.
- Practicing or sharing information on cultural humility (e.g. toileting practices among Muslim clients).
- Starting a journal club on issues related to DEI+.
- Holding a "culture education" day to share information about various cultures and ethnicities and how that affects daily function and OT practice (e.g. discussing Shabbat practices in an inpatient rehabilitation unit).

- Starting a diverse guest speaker series by inviting colleagues from other areas to talk about their take on DEI+ issues (e.g. the effect of language barriers in non-English-speaking clients and adherence to treatment).
- Establishing collaborations with academic institutions to stay connected with OT/OTA students on DEI+ issues (e.g. student-led organizations).
- Connecting with the state or local OT associations to foster DEI+ initiatives and collaboration in an area of practice.

Professional development, engagement, and DEI+

Similar to others in healthcare professions, occupational therapy students transitioning to the clinic must acquire a lifelong learning approach to maintain their clinical and professional competence. For example, to maintain board certification and state licensure students must pursue opportunities for continuing education (i.e. activities that enhance clinical knowledge and skills) and professional development (i.e. activities that enhance professional, interprofessional, and leadership skills). Additionally, students may pursue local and national and preferably international professional engagement opportunities (i.e. activities that enhance skills of networking, advocacy, and volunteering) to enhance the caliber of their professional profile and connection to their communities.

While professional development is meant to amplify clinicians' careers, the majority of pursued activities are typically geared to advancing practical aspects of the job (e.g. program evaluation, supervisory roles) with less focus on issues related to DEI+ (e.g. social drivers of health affecting the client). This may unfortunately increase the gap between clinical practices and DEI+ issues inherent in the communities and affecting the clients. Professional engagement is a space for learning, understanding, and addressing DEI+ that may be overlooked with the typical activities pursued in the professional development agenda.

Intentionally pursuing professional engagement activities that revolve around DEI+ within the surrounding community may fill in the gap for DEI+. For example, when practitioners engage with local community-based organizations they become aware of socio-eco-political issues affecting their local clients (e.g. learning the existing needs of local families in marginalized communities with no health insurance).

The activities listed below are a few examples of professional engagement activities that can enhance practitioners' understanding of the nexus between DEI+ issues and clinical practice. Note how these activities are not typically considered professional development activities for many practicing occupational therapists.

- Connecting with various local faith-based organizations to understand the role of faith, spirituality, mindfulness, and religious practices in daily activities.
- Engaging with disability volunteer and advocacy groups to explore initiatives enhancing accessibilities for practitioners, students, and clients with disabilities.
- Using social media to connect with social advocacy groups to increase outreach to community-based supporters and advocates.
- Establishing outreach to school districts serving underserved communities to increase the visibility of OT services to marginalized or overlooked communities (e.g. refugee children).
- Participating in open community-based events (e.g. fundraisers, cultural weeks, food festivals) to expand exposure to various ethnographic communities.

CASE EXAMPLE 8.2: Fares and Hana hold a multi-faith panel

Fares and Hana are two new practitioners in a large hospital in an urban area. The two met during the onboarding process and got to work together on several cases. Several months later during one of the team social events, the new practitioners start talking about their ethnic and faith backgrounds (Muslim and Jewish) and notice that others on the team held several misconceptions about both religions. Fares and Hana decide to organize a panel on the intersectionality of religion and clinical practice to share information about their ethno-religious backgrounds, and invite questions about clinical implications when dealing with clients of these faith groups. During the panel, the practitioners talk about religious observations and practices that affect daily activities (e.g. prayers, fasting, Shabbat, major holidays throughout the year, dietary restrictions based on religion).

Reflective pause

- What do you think of the panel discussion the new practitioners introduce to the team?
- What is the value of highlighting faith in a clinical setting?
- How do you think others on the team will respond to the panel and why?

Commentary on Case example 8.2

This scenario describes a professional engagement activity that is geared toward DEI+. Ethnic and religious backgrounds are usually overlooked in clinical practice due to the complex and private nature of constructs of religion, spirituality, and ethnic traditions. Research shows that practitioners' religious and spiritual orientation can positively impact clinical practice with various clients (Palmer Kelly *et al.*, 2020). Such activity by Fares and Hana not only highlights a central construct in clinical practice but also sheds light on the practitioner's intersectionality and how that may influence their approach to their work experience. While some colleagues may find value in such a panel, others may not prioritize learning about this aspect of DEI+. Practitioners should not be discouraged by others' responses or attitudes toward professional engagement activities such as the one described in the scenario.

The first year as an occupational therapy practitioner

Multiple factors surrounding the practice area, such as the setting, location, and funding, can result in DEI+ initiatives not being prioritized in daily practice and clinical research (El-Galaly *et al.*, 2023; Johnson *et al.*, 2024). Exploring culturally variant daily activities and culturally relevant assessment tools, and enhancing accessibility measures for clients and practitioners, are a few common examples of overlooked DEI+ initiatives (Feldner *et al.*, 2022; Muñoz, 2007). Reasons for that may be outside the control of the practitioner, such as the mission of the institution, uncommunicated agendas by business owners (e.g. unspoken ideology), or simply insufficient time and resources to support DEI+. Regardless of the circumstances surrounding their practice, DEI+ mindful practitioners must identify clear goals for their professional transformation. In fact, during the first year as an OTP, you should identify a list of multifaceted goals as a clinician. These goals should include practice goals (e.g. diversifying clinical expertise), professional goals (e.g. inter-professional events), and professional engagement goals (e.g. connecting with local communities). To support any or all of these goals, new practitioners may benefit from the checklist below for useful things they can do or commit to during their first year

- Seek mentorship or guidance on professional development and engagement goals.
- Seek and provide peer support to enhance clinical and professional practice.
- Join support groups for DEI+-related issues such as affinity or advocacy groups.
- Consult with or start a caring community (i.e. groups that provide support and enhance a sense of belonging) (Suarez-Balcazar *et al.*, 2023).
- Join the state OT association and attend their meetings.
- Join the national OT association (American Occupational Therapy Association) and engage in their community of practice.
- Establish or join a journal club to boost your evidence-based practice skills. One recommendation would be finding the established Clinical Practice Guideline Publications by AOTA in your area of practice.
- Establish a social group to enhance self-care and social well-being with peers.

CASE EXAMPLE 8.3: "Jade, you speak like a White girl!"

Jade starts her first job as an occupational therapy assistant in a private practice owned by a physical therapist. Jade grew up in a suburban area that is predominantly White in New Jersey. Jade is bilingual and speaks Creole fluently because of her Haitian heritage. A few days after she starts, her supervisor, who identifies as a White male, asks her where she is originally from. She answers that she is from Long Branch, New Jersey. The supervisor stares at Jade for a few seconds and then asks, "Where are you originally from?" Jade answers that she is Haitian, to which he responds, "Interesting, you speak English like a White girl." Jade does not answer. Although Jade is very upset with that comment, she decides to address the issue at a later time, fearing to create tension early in her career.

Reflective pause

- What do you think of the comment the supervisor makes? Is it a compliment?
- What is the right response to the supervisor's comment?
- What should Jade do in this scenario?

Commentary on Case example 8.3

This scenario is a classic example of microaggressions that practitioners of color face during their daily practice. Although Jade is a vocal and strong advocate of DEI+, such issues may be more intimidating at work given the complicated things at stake, such as career progression, job security, power dynamics, and collegial interaction. No matter how difficult the scenario is, Jade has options to address that interaction. One option is asking a trusted colleague for advice, consulting with human resources (if confidentiality is guaranteed), or speaking directly with the supervisor. Albeit prohibited in the laws of equal employment opportunities, retaliation exists in many cases, especially against people of color (Snipe, 2024). Practitioners of color must seek resources to help them navigate incidents of discrimination and microaggressions in the workplace, especially early in their careers. Additionally, all practitioners must select a time and place for addressing such comments to ensure their work safety and professional well-being. Jade could address the issue at a later time when she has gathered some ideas to safely navigate this incident (e.g. brainstorm with leaders in the field or with colleagues with experience in microaggressions).

DEI+, allies, advocates, and accomplices, and culture change: How does the journey continue?

Occupational therapy students should understand that being allies, advocates, and accomplices in social justice is essential for their professional work and personal development. This commitment goes beyond mere compliance with ethical standards; it fosters a deeper understanding of the social determinants of health and the structural inequalities that affect their clients. By actively engaging in social justice, occupational therapy students can enhance their empathy and cultural humility, which are critical for delivering client-centered care. This engagement helps them recognize the unique challenges faced by marginalized populations and empowers them to address these challenges through tailored interventions and advocacy efforts (Muldoon, 2022).

Being an ally in the field of occupational therapy means standing in solidarity with marginalized groups and acknowledging the privilege one holds. Allies use their positions to amplify the voices of those who are often unheard, ensuring that their clients' needs and perspectives are respected and valued. This role involves continuous self-reflection and education about issues such as racism, sexism, ableism, and other forms of discrimination. For occupational therapy students, this means actively seeking out resources, attending workshops, and participating in discussions that enhance their understanding of these issues. By doing so, they prepare themselves to create inclusive environments that promote equity in healthcare settings (Djulus *et al.*, 2021).

Advocacy in occupational therapy extends beyond individual client interactions to systemic change. Students should learn to identify and challenge policies and practices that perpetuate health disparities. This can involve lobbying for legislation that improves access to occupational therapy services, participating in professional organizations that promote social justice, and engaging in community outreach programs. Advocacy efforts not only benefit clients but also advance the profession by positioning occupational therapists as leaders in the movement for equitable healthcare. By developing these advocacy skills, students can contribute to a more just and inclusive healthcare system.

Accompliceship takes allyship and advocacy a step further by actively dismantling oppressive systems. This role requires occupational therapy students to use their knowledge and skills to create tangible change. Accomplices work alongside marginalized communities, taking direction from those directly affected by injustice. In practice, this could involve collaborating with community organizations to develop programs that address specific needs, conducting research that highlights disparities and solutions, or mentoring peers from underrepresented backgrounds. Being an accomplice means committing to long-term, sustained efforts to achieve social justice, recognizing that this work is crucial for the well-being of all clients.

Incorporating these roles into their professional identity enables occupational therapy students to develop a holistic approach to care. Understanding and addressing the broader context in which clients live enhances therapeutic outcomes and ensures that interventions are relevant and effective. For example, the occupational therapy student can integrate aspects of the physical, digital, cultural, and temporal context as a means to better understand how a multifaceted context impacts the therapeutic process as well as the impact of disability on daily activities. Furthermore, this commitment to social justice fosters professional growth, as students learn to navigate complex social dynamics and advocate for systemic change. Ultimately, being allies, advocates, and accomplices in social justice enriches the practice of occupational therapy, ensuring that it remains a compassionate, inclusive, and equitable profession.

CASE EXAMPLE 8.4: Ashwayna runs for state board elections
Ashwayna (Ash) is an alumnus of the program and is a passionate school-based practitioner. She enjoys working with her students and especially seeing their progress outside school as she runs a community-based program for students transitioning to vocational settings. She is an avid advocate within her practice setting and has even set out advocacy rallies for greater inclusion of mental health within pediatric practice. Ash, as she is known by her friends, notices a social media post for her state occupational therapy association requesting nominations for board positions. Ash commits to learning more about this and notices that there are no pediatric or school-based clinicians on the board and that school-based practice is a large employment setting within her state. Ash spends days contemplating whether she has what it takes to fulfill the duties of the position and even has a sense of being an imposter based on the way she feels about herself, stating, "Will they even know how to pronounce my name? I don't even have as much experience as the current board members." Ash does not know what to do but has an undeniable urge to do something, especially in advocacy, for her practice, and practices within under-served areas of need.

Reflective pause

- Why would Ash be experiencing imposter syndrome and does it happen to everyone?
- Who should Ash seek support from and why?
- What would happen if Ash decides to not pursue this opportunity and will it further impact how she feels about herself?

Commentary on Case example 8.4

Ash is not alone. There are countless reasons why she may be feeling under-confident about the current opportunity at hand, an opportunity to serve and incite change through active leadership; however, it's also a clear challenge that requires Ash to self-reflect and embrace the need for support. Stepping out of the student role and into the shoes of a clinician is not an easy task, nor is it a static process. Many practitioners admit that being a student is an incredible opportunity to actualize the type of practitioner you want to strive towards, and that the drive for learning never truly ends. Ash is in a space within her professional journey where she is torn between self-doubt and trust. Individuals relating to Ash or experiencing similar situations that can include opportunities within their academic programs, employment opportunities, and advocacy roles in community spaces must remember the importance of mentorship, which in itself is a dynamic and ever-changing process of self-discovery, community building, and humility.

DEI+ and the next generations of occupational therapy students

Occupational therapy practitioners offer invaluable advice to future students through the lens of diversity, equity, and inclusion. First, they emphasize the importance of cultural humility. Future occupational therapists should strive to understand and respect the diverse backgrounds, beliefs, and values of their clients. This requires continuous self-education and reflection to recognize their own biases and assumptions. Practitioners advise students to actively seek out opportunities to engage with diverse communities, whether through volunteering, internships, or participating in cultural humility training. By doing so, students can build the empathy and understanding necessary to provide truly client-centered care that respects and honors each individual's unique context.

Moreover, practitioners stress the need for advocacy in promoting equity within the occupational therapy profession and the broader healthcare system. They encourage students to become involved in professional organizations and community initiatives that address health disparities and promote social justice. This involvement can take many forms, such as lobbying for policy changes, participating in research that highlights inequities, or educating peers and colleagues about DEI+ issues. By being proactive advocates, future occupational therapists can help ensure that all individuals, regardless of their background, have access to high-quality, equitable healthcare services. This advocacy not only benefits clients but also strengthens the profession by demonstrating its commitment to justice and inclusivity.

Additionally, occupational therapy practitioners highlight the significance of creating inclusive environments within educational and clinical settings. They advise students to foster a culture of inclusion where diverse perspectives are valued and everyone feels respected and supported. This involves actively listening to and collaborating with clients, colleagues, and community members from diverse backgrounds. Practitioners recommend that students develop strong communication and interpersonal skills, which are essential for building trust and rapport with clients from various walks of life. By embracing inclusivity, future occupational therapists can enhance their ability to address the unique needs of each client, ultimately improving therapeutic outcomes and contributing to a more equitable society.

> **CASE EXAMPLE 8.5:** Allie and Gemma meet
> with the new students and share the lessons
> learned during their OT studies
>
> Allie and Gemma are thrilled to have the opportunity to share their lived experiences and foster a greater sense of belonging for the new cohort through holding an informal meet and greet! Allie is passionate about creating a mentor/mentee program that allows individuals to feel connected and supported, and most importantly to be a part of a community, and she is planning on disseminating a survey that allows new and current students to connect on deeper levels. Gemma is working on a presentation that also supports new students in building a sense of community and embracing belonging through opening up various channels of dialogue and support systems, both within and external to the program. It will also provide opportunities for new students to connect with the faculty as organically and authentically as possible.
>
> As Allie and Gemma prepare to deliver their presentation to the new cohort, they pause to give each other space to express their stories, recognize their growth both personally and professionally, and cherish how much they've experienced together as developing practitioners and friends. They recognize that the experiences within their program are not exclusive to them and that they reflect the stories of

countless others who may be experiencing challenges and barriers to education, practice, and advocacy. They acknowledge that opening a space to lean into the uncomfortable is the first step in embracing sustainable change.

Reflective pause

- Are there any creative forms of mentorship you've experienced personally or professionally and how has this impacted your life?
- If there was a single message you could give yourself when entering the program, what would it be and why?
- As an occupational therapy student within a cohort of peers, is growth and embracing experiences more meaningful when experienced and shared by a collective? Why or why not?

Commentary on Case example 8.5

The transition from student to clinician happens on day one within your program. Embracing that you are just as much a part of the occupational therapy community as any other stakeholder is the first step in your journey to growth, change, and advocacy. Allie and Gemma are symbols of occupational therapy students who look both inward and outward for the change they want to see, especially for those who cannot see it themselves. Allyship and peer-mentorship are critical aspects of any professional program and extend to lessons learned both in and out of the classroom. Challenging yourself as a student to take on responsibilities, to be there for others through student associations and community-based activities, is one of many ways to feel connected to those you serve, through both empathy and accountability. Whether it's an activity you develop outside your primary fieldwork roles, an expanded way to connect with individuals within under-served communities through a master's project, or an innovative way to match occupational therapy services to unmet areas of need through a capstone initiative, the growth and impact of occupational therapy is boundless and only heightened by your untapped potential.

Let's think about it

Gemma notices a call for proposals for an upcoming conference and is very excited, nervous, and anxious about this opportunity to share the amazing data collected from her community-based project that she has been working on since she was in OT school. Gemma submits a proposal and anxiously waits for a response from the peer-reviewed committee. After several weeks, Gemma receives an email from the conference team, and it is not what she was expecting. Her proposal is denied, and the email provides peer-reviewed feedback and suggested areas of improvement. Gemma is crushed and now feels insecure about her work and is contemplating whether she should still go to the conference.

Gemma decides to submit to the state conference later in the year. She later finds out that her proposal is accepted. She is excited to take part in her first annual conference as a new practitioner. She has already requested time off from work, has set up her cases to ensure that there is adequate coverage, and has even created mini-case studies of her current clients to ensure that the covering provider is abreast of the progress and ongoing needs. Gemma successfully presents at the conference, recalling funny short tips and tricks from Dr. Campbell and Dr. Cruz when she was in the program on how to ensure that the way you practice OT is just as neat and organized as your shoe closet!

A few weeks after her presentation, Gemma meets Allie for lunch to talk about the conference and the people she met during the conference events. The two start planning a joint proposal for the next national annual conference.

Recap

As students and new practitioners venture into the roles of clinicians and professionals, it is important to remember that this line of professional growth is non-linear. Activities such as presenting at a professional conference can have some challenges such as preparing proposals, presenting, and securing travel funding. The effort and cost of such activities can be overwhelming but the benefits of this kind of professional adventure are rewarding, with various career enhancement opportunities such as networking, professional visibility, collaboration, and overall professional advancement.

Reflective thinking

- How do you handle disappointment, and should it be in the same manner professionally?

Critical thinking

- Is sharing your work, passion, and interests at any professional conference a form of advocacy? Why or why not?

Action-oriented thinking

- What steps can Gemma take to learn from this situation, both personally and professionally?

HOT TAKE

Which one is more important, job stability or professional well-being? Should we address bias and microaggressions in the workplace?

Suggested reading to navigate this question: "Professionalism: Microaggressions in the healthcare setting" (Ehie *et al.*, 2021)

References

Djulus, G., Sheikhan, N. Y., Nawaz, E., Burley, J., *et al.* (2021). Advancing allyship through anti-oppression workshops for public health students: A mixed methods pilot evaluation. *Pedagogy in Health Promotion, 7*(4), 304–312. https://doi.org/10.1177/23733799209624l0

Ehie, O., Muse, I., Hill, L., & Bastien, A. (2021). Professionalism: Microaggression in the healthcare setting. *Current Opinion in Anaesthesiology, 34*(2), 131–136. https://doi.org/10.1097/ACO.0000000000000966

El-Galaly, T. C., Gaidzik, V. I., Gaman, M.-A., Antic, D., *et al.* and on behalf of the EHA Diversity, Equity, and Inclusion Taskforce. (2023). A lack of diversity, equity, and inclusion in clinical research has a direct impact on patient care. *HemaSphere, 7*(3), e842. https://doi.org/10.1097/HS9.0000000000000842

Feldner, H. A., Evans, H. D., Chamblin, K., Ellis, L. M., *et al.* (2022). Infusing disability equity within rehabilitation education and practice: A qualitative study of lived experiences of ableism, allyship, and healthcare partnership. *Frontiers in Rehabilitation Sciences, 3,* 947592. https://doi.org/10.3389/fresc.2022.947592

Johnson, K. R., Washington, S. E., Hoyt, C. R., Banks, T. M., Román-Oyola, R., & Hamed, R. (2024). Establishing diversity, equity, and inclusion priorities for occupational therapy research. *American Journal of Occupational Therapy, 78*(1), 7801349010. https://doi.org/10.5014/ajot.2024.050601

Moir, E. M. A., Turpin, M. J., & Copley, J. A. (2021). The clinical challenges experienced by new graduate occupational therapists: A matrix review. *Canadian Journal of Occupational Therapy, 88*(3), 200–213. https://doi.org/10.1177/0008417421I022880

Muldoon, K. M. (2022). Improving communication about diversity, equity, and inclusion in health professions education. *The Anatomical Record, 305*(4), 1000–1018. https://doi.org/10.1002/ar.24864

Muñoz, J. P. (2007). Culturally responsive caring in occupational therapy. *Occupational Therapy International, 14*(4), Article 4. https://doi.org/10.1002/oti.238

Opoku, E. N., Khuabi, L.-A. J.-N., & Van Niekerk, L. (2021). Exploring the factors that affect the transition from student to health professional: An integrative review. *BMC Medical Education, 21*(1), 558. https://doi.org/10.1186/s12909-021-02978-0

Palmer Kelly, E., Hyer, M., Payne, N., & Pawlik, T. M. (2020). Does spiritual and religious orientation impact the clinical practice of healthcare providers? *Journal of Interprofessional Care, 34*(4), 520–527. https://doi.org/10.1080/13561820.2019.1709426

Picotin, J., Beaudoin, M., Hélie, S., Martin, A.-É., & Carrier, A. (2021). Occupational therapists as social change agents: Exploring factors that influence their actions. *Canadian Journal of Occupational Therapy, 88*(3), 231–243. https://doi.org/10.1177/00084174211022891

Snipe, M. (2024). Health care workers are speaking up about the racism in facilities nationwide. *Capital B.* https://capitalbnews.org/health-care-industry-racism

Suarez-Balcazar, Y., Arias, D., & Muñoz, J. P. (2023). Promoting justice, diversity, equity, and inclusion through caring communities: Why it matters to occupational therapy. *American Journal of Occupational Therapy, 77*(6), 7706347020. https://doi.org/10.5014/ajot.2023.050416

Appendix 1: Characters Across the Book Chapters

See character matrix in Appendix 2 for more details about each character.

Chapter 1	Chapter 2	Chapter 3	Chapter 4
Allie	Allie	Allie	Malik
Gemma	Gemma	Gemma	Jamie
Dr. Boyle	Amihan	Dr. Boyle	Christopher
Memona	Cheyenne	Dr. Gallagher	Dr. Campbell
Amihan	Malik	Yara	
Julian	Dr. Campbell	Elizabeth	
Israa	Dr. Taylor	Cheyenne	
	Dr. Klein	Hana	
	Dr. Singh	Dr. Moore	
	Dr. Cruz		

Chapter 5	Chapter 6	Chapter 7	Chapter 8
Allie	Dr. Taylor	Allie	Allie
Gemma	Malik	Gemma	Gemma
Memona	Christopher	Lauren	Fares
Dr. Boyle	Elizabeth	Cheyenne	Hana
Dr. Campbell	Jennie	Israa	Ashwayna (Ash)
Levi		Lin	Dr. Campbell
		Dr. Boyle	Dr. Cruz
		Dr. Joseph	Jade
		Dr. Klein	

Appendix 2: Character Matrix

Character name and role	Some layers of intersectional diversity		Character highlights
Allie (she/her) Entry-level Master of Occupational Therapy (MOT) student in an occupational therapy program in an urban city in the North East. Originally from the North East region	**Race:** White-Italian **GI:** Cis female **Ethnicity:** Non-Hispanic **SES:** Upper middle class	**SO:** Heterosexual **Ability/ disability:** Dyslexia **Faith:** Catholic, Christian	Identifies as an extrovert, ally, vocal about social justice, supportive family, and network of friends. Allie had a transgender cousin who died by suicide after incidents of bullying and a diagnosis of depression and substance use. She is a strong advocate against bullying and bias in her local community.
Gemma (she/her) Entry-level MOT occupational therapy program in an urban city in the North East. Originally from the South region	**Race:** Black-Latina **GI:** Cis female **Ethnicity:** Hispanic **SES:** Middle class	**SO:** Heterosexual **Ability/ disability:** Diabetes type I **Faith:** Catholic	Identifies as an introvert and first generation, experiences bias and microaggressions toward her race, and advocates for social justice, equity, and inclusion. Bilingual. Has a sibling with a physical disability who uses a wheelchair for mobility and activities of daily living.
Israa (she/her) Entry-level MOT student currently in fieldwork Level II. Family from Eygpt, born in the United States	**Race:** White-North African **GI:** Cis female **Ethnicity:** Non-Hispanic **SES:** Lower middle class	**SO:** Heterosexual **Ability/ disability:** Myopia (short-sightedness) **Faith:** Muslim (Hijabi: wears head cover)	Quiet, supportive, experiences bias and microaggressions toward her faith as Muslim. Advocates for social justice. Bilingual.

Elizabeth (she/they) Entry-level MOT student	**Race:** White-Irish **GI:** Cis female **Ethnicity:** Non-Hispanic **SES:** Lower middle class	**SO:** Queer **Ability/disability:** Anxiety **Faith:** Agnostic	Identifies as introvert, critical, vegan, environmentalist, feminist.
Amihan (she/they) Entry-level MOT student from San Diego, California	**Race:** Asian-Filipino **GI:** Cis female **Ethnicity:** Non-Hispanic **SES:** Upper middle class	**SO:** Queer **Ability/disability:** ADHD and eating disorder **Faith:** Catholic Christian	Identifies as second generation, self-described as obese, and faces cultural stigma for her weight and sexual orientation. Receives testing accommodations. Bilingual.
Jennie (she/her) Entry-level MOT student from Washington State	**Race:** Asian-Korean **GI:** Cis female **Ethnicity:** Non-Hispanic **SES:** Upper middle class	**SO:** Heterosexual **Ability/disability:** None **Faith:** Christian	An only child, has a small family, supportive of classmates, bilingual.
Christopher (he/his) Entry-level OTD student	**Race:** Mixed race (Haitian-Mexican) **GI:** Cis male **Ethnicity:** Hispanic **SES:** Lower middle class	**SO:** Heterosexual **Ability/disability:** None **Faith:** Catholic Christian	Identifies as first generation, single parent who works two part-time jobs to support the family.
Hana (she/her) Entry-level MOT student (Chapter 3) and new practitioner (Chapter 8)	**Race:** White **GI:** Cis female **Ethnicity:** Non-Hispanic **SES:** Lower middle class	**SO:** Heterosexual **Ability/disability:** Learning disability **Faith:** Orthodox Jewish	Receives testing accommodation, friendly, hardworking student, quiet in class.
Levi (they/them) Entry-level MOT student originally from North East area	**Race:** White **GI:** Trans woman **Ethnicity:** Non-Hispanic **SES:** Upper middle class	**SO:** bisexual **Ability/disability:** Anxiety **Faith:** Christian	Expressed concerns about the application forms in the admission process. They also had a few instances of being misgendered by their peers and faculty members.

Character name and role	Some layers of intersectional diversity		Character highlights
Cheyenne (she/her) Entry-level MOT student	**Race:** Indigenous **GI:** Cis female **Ethnicity:** Non-Hispanic **SES:** Lower middle class	**SO:** Heterosexual **Ability/disability:** Treated for mild depressive symptoms **Faith:** Spiritual/Washani	Identifies as first generation college student, advocate for Indigenous heritage and culture. Supportive of classmates, identifies as non-confrontational.
Fares (he/him) New OT practitioner	**Race:** White-Middle Eastern **GI:** Cis male **Ethnicity:** Arab non-Hispanic **SES:** Upper middle class	**SO:** Heterosexual **Ability/disability:** Hearing impairment **Faith:** Muslim (Shia)	Advocate for Arab and Muslim culture in the workplace, supportive of co-workers and clients.
Memona (she/her) MOT student	**Race:** South Asian **GI:** Cis female **Ethnicity:** Pakistani **SES:** Lower middle class	**SO:** Prefers not to disclose **Ability/disability:** Chronic autoimmune disease **Faith:** Islam (Sunni)	She is an observant Muslim and is experiencing difficulty with bullying from her peers due to her faith-based garments. She also has an accent and her peers find it difficult to understand her at times.
Jamie (they/them) Entry-level OTD student	**Race:** White **Ethnicity:** Irish non-Hispanic **GI:** Cis female **SES:** Upper middle class	**SO:** Homosexual **Ability/disability:** Self-disclosed bipolar **Faith:** Catholic	Wants to be liked by everyone and makes it a priority to connect with peers and faculty, often in an aggressive fashion. Is often labeled intrusive and opportunistic within social interactions.
Julian (he/his) Occupational therapy assistant student	**Race:** Mixed race **GI:** Cis male **Ethnicity:** Hispanic **SES:** Lower middle class	**SO:** Heterosexual **Ability/disability:** Physical disability, uses a cane **Faith:** Catholic	Works while in the program and is often difficult to reach by his peers for group assignments or social engagements. Supports his family and is the primary breadwinner.
Yara (she/her) MOT student	**Race:** North African **GI:** Cis female **Ethnicity:** Moroccan-Arab, non-Hispanic **SES:** Upper middle class	**SO:** Heterosexual **Ability/disability:** None **Faith:** Muslim	Yara is a second generation Arab who identifies as Muslim. Active in advocacy on social justice issues.

Malik (he/him) Entry-level OTD student	**Race:** Black **GI:** Cis male **Ethnicity:** Non-Hispanic **SES:** Lower middle class	**SO:** Heterosexual **Ability/ disability:** None **Faith:** Protestant	Highly intelligent but has never traveled much due to his SES. Looking to further himself and change "the cycle" for his family and the community. Is a positive change-maker in his community.
Ashwayna (Ash) (she/her) Alumnus of the MOT program	**Race:** South Asian **GI:** Cis female **Ethnicity:** Bengali non-Hispanic **SES:** Lower middle class	**SO:** Heterosexual **Ability/ disability:** None **Faith:** Hindu	Serves on the alumni council for her program. Active in areas of leadership and advocacy.
Jade (she/her) Occupational therapy assistant	**Race:** Black **GI:** Cis female **Ethnicity:** Haitian, non-Hispanic **SES:** Lower middle class	**SO:** Heterosexual **Ability/ disability:** None **Faith:** Protestant	A strong advocate for DEI+ in her school and community. Attends advocacy events by local and national OT association.
Lauren (she/her) Fieldwork II educator with three years of clinical experience	**Race:** White-Polish **GI:** Cis female **Ethnicity:** Non-Hispanic **SES:** Middle class	**SO:** Heterosexual **Ability/ disability:** None **Faith:** Baptist	Graduated from a large university in the Midwest region and moved to the North East five years ago.
Dr. Klein (she/her) Joint Academic Fieldwork Coordinator for two small cohorts (MOT and OTD)	**Race:** White **GI:** Cis female **Ethnicity:** Non-Hispanic **SES:** Upper middle class	**SO:** Heterosexual **Ability/ disability:** Spinal cord injury—uses a wheelchair for mobility **Faith:** Jewish	Supportive of students in fieldwork, with 20 years of experience in the field. Expresses experiencing anti-semitic incidents in the clinic and as a former student. Advocates for accessibility issues in educational and clinical spaces.
Dr. Cruz (she/her) Program Director	**Race:** White (Cuban) **GI:** Cis female **Ethnicity:** Hispanic American **SES:** Upper middle class	**SO:** Not disclosed **Ability/ disability:** None **Faith:** Catholic	Experienced program director who oversees two educational programs, and has held multiple leadership positions. Identifies as a conservative educator who prioritizes program affairs over extracurricular activities.

Character name and role	Some layers of intersectional diversity		Character highlights
Dr. Campbell (she/her) Full-time faculty in multiple OT programs. Teaches physical dysfunctions, advocacy, leadership	Race: Black GI: Cis female Ethnicity: Jamaican, non-Hispanic SES: Upper middle class	SO: Heterosexual Ability/ disability: None Faith: Christian	Jamaican American who is proud of her Caribbean roots. Supportive of and identifies publicly as Black and supports American Black culture, but is still learning to understand US dynamics. She strongly identifies with Caribbean culture, which is not always respected by others.
Dr. Taylor (xe/xem) Full-time faculty, teaches modules on physical disabilities and neurosciences	Race: Black GI: Cis male Ethnicity: Non-Hispanic SES: Lower middle class	SO: Homosexual Ability/ disability: None Faith: Baptist	Engaging faculty member who believes in inclusive teaching and learning spaces. Known for xyr sense of humor and support for students. Runs affinity groups for students of color who identify as members of the LGBTQ community.
Dr. Boyle (she/her) Full-time faculty teaches psychosocial courses, administration, and community capstones (MS and OTD students)	Race: White GI: Cis female Ethnicity: Non-Hispanic SES: Upper middle class	SO: Heterosexual Ability/ disability: Breast cancer survivor with mild lymphedema in her left arm Faith: Protestant Christian	Identifies as an introvert, non-confrontational, and supports students of all diverse backgrounds. She is a firm believer in inter-professional collaboration in OT and the need for professional and networking skills for career success. Does a lot of volunteering work for the local church in her community.
Dr. Moore (she/her) Full-time faculty: theory, activity analysis, introduction to OT	Race: White GI: Cis female Ethnicity: Hispanic (Puerto Rican) SES: Upper middle class	SO: Heterosexual Ability/ disability: None Faith: Catholic Christian	Supportive of students, and faculty advisor for student-run organizations. Bilingual.

Dr. Gallagher (she/her) Fieldwork coordinator at an MOT program. Full-time faculty, teaches kinesiology	Race: White-Irish GI: Cis female Ethnicity: Non-Hispanic SES: Upper middle class	SO: Heterosexual Ability/ disability: Non-disclosed Faith: Jewish	Supportive of students in fieldwork experiences but believes that students should work with fieldwork educators to improve their clinical skills and incorporate their feedback even if they disagree with it. Believes that all fieldwork educators are supportive of students but the newer generations are less resilient compared to her generation of students.
Dr. Singh (he/him) Full-time faculty, teaches anatomy	Race: Brown GI: Cis male Ethnicity: South Asian, non-Hispanic SES: Lower middle class	SO: Heterosexual Ability/ disability: None Faith: Hindu	An assistant professor who migrated from India with his family a few years ago. He is friendly and works very well with students who describe him as very supportive and respectful of all students. He has an Indian accent.
Dr. Joseph (she/her) Doctoral capstone coordinator	Race: White GI: Cis female Ethnicity: Non-Hispanic SES: Upper middle class	SO: Heterosexual Ability/ disability: None Faith: Catholic Christian	Supports students during their capstones. Described as friendly.

Note: SO = sexual orientation; SES = socioeconomic status; GI = gender identity

About the Authors

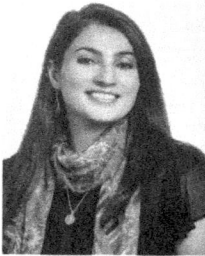

Dr. Razan Hamed PhD., OTR/L, FAOTA (she/her) is a cis-gendered female who serves as Associate Professor and Associate Director of the Programs in Occupational Therapy (CUOT) at Columbia University. In this book, Dr. Hamed uses her intersectional experiences as a woman of color of Arab descent, an academician, and a leader in the field of occupational therapy. Dr. Hamed is an advocate for issues related to DEI+ in occupational therapy education and clinical and professional practice. Her experiences are also inspired by her former roles as a member of the Inaugural American Occupational Therapy Association DEI+ Committee, and the founder of the Arab American Occupational Therapy Group, and her teaching experiences on DEI+ issues. Dr. Hamed is a firm believer in the power of empathetic conversations and culturally mindful practices in overcoming bias in our society and in occupational therapy.

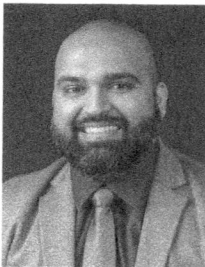

Dr. Vikram Pagpatan EdD, OTR/L, FAOTA (he/him) is a cis-gendered male. Dr. Pagpatan is of Asian-American descent and practices in academia and pediatrics within New York State. DEI+ through Dr. Pagpatan's lived experiences symbolizes a society that practices tolerance and reflection of topics, communities, and thoughts that thread all of us together. Dr. Pagpatan has previously served on the AOTA DEI Committee, is the immediate past President of the Association of Asian-Americans and Pacific Islanders in Occupational Therapy and is a board director for the American Occupational Therapy Association, and has authored several textbooks for the profession. Dr. Pagpatan's vision for this text is to inspire those in the room to remain in the room with confidence and inspiration.

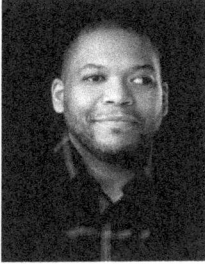

Mr. André Johnson MS, OTR/L, COTA/L, ROH (he/him) is a cis-gendered male. Mr. Johnson practices in pediatrics, orthopedics, and academia in Florida. In this book, Mr. Johnson uses his intersectional experiences as a Black male of American, Jamaican, Chinese, and Cuban descent, while being a practitioner, academician, and leader in occupational therapy. Mr. Johnson advocates for authenthic DEI+ effort and threads it into his clinical practice as an occupational therapy assistant and educator. Mr. Johnson has previously served as Chairperson of the AOTA Commission on Education, Vice President of the Black-male Registered Occupational Therapy Healthcare-professionals Assistants & Students (BROTHAS) organization, and is currently a Board Director for the American Occupational Therapy Association. He is a firm believer in the power of connection and that every individual has the responsibility, energy, and ability to make a difference in society and the occupational therapy profession.

DEI+ Workbook: Structured Exercises and Discussion Prompts

How to use this workbook

This workbook provides additional opportunities for students to reflect on the content provided in the chapters. It solidifies their understanding of how issues related to DEI+ impact their interactions with others during their professional and clinical practices.

The content of this workbook can be used after reading each chapter (recommended) or after reading the entire book. It is recommended that the exercises be facilitated by someone who is not participating in the dialogue (e.g. an educator, teaching assistant, student leader) to provide an objective perspective. These exercises can also be used as a springboard for panel discussions, student-led activities of events, or for ideas for guest speakers to address. The content was designed in this format to allow the exercises to be used in an educational (e.g. assigned by the educators), professional (e.g. addressed by guest speakers), or collegial (e.g. used by student leadership groups) context.

This workbook contains eight worksheets that correspond to each chapter in the book. The exercises provided in each sheet are systematically created to improve skills related to active and accurate listening, perspective sharing, and empathetic interactions. Each worksheet provides the following:

1. **Role-play exercise:** To enhance perspective-sharing and communication skills. These exercises help in learning, relearning, or

unlearning untested perspectives about others, including conceptions that are based on implicit bias and stereotypes.

2. **Debate team:** Exercises to offer an open forum for students to create and deliver arguments supported by evidence, expert opinions, or lived experiences on issues related to DEI+ in education and professional and clinical practice. These exercises enhance students' skills to create valid points for building perspective, advocating for oneself and others, and challenging biased actions.

3. **Action-oriented:** Suggestions to prompt students to identify actionable behaviors that can support their point of view or challenge a biased perspective. These actions can also be geared toward advocating for oneself, the client, or other individuals or communities related to occupational therapy practice.

Diversity, Equity, Inclusion and Other Aspects of Social Justice (DEI+)

1. **Role play:** Describe a common scenario related to the chapter, with the students taking different perspectives on issues. Determine how many students are involved in this scenario. Describe the context in as much detail as needed.

   - Goal: To encourage students to share perspectives and lived experiences.

   - Example: Two students with different backgrounds applying to the same OT program.

2. **Debate team:** Describe a controversial issue and encourage students to read an article, seek opinions, or compose an argument to discuss the issue from different perspectives.

   - Goal: To promote allyship, advocacy, and leadership.

   - Example: Citing one article, extracting a quote, and highlighting a historical event such as state laws on DEI+.

3. **Take action:** Describe an action students must take to serve a goal relevant to the objectives of the chapter.

   - Goal: Enhance students' skills to take tangible actions to promote or serve issues related to DEI+ in their education and early clinical practice.

   - Examples: Write a letter to a legislator to introduce a bill supporting OT services for underserved populations; meet with students from other schools with a different OT degree (e.g. OTA, OTD, EdD).

Allyship, Accompliceship, and Advocacy: How Can I Help?

1. **Role play:** Describe a moral dilemma related to the chapter, with the students taking a definitive perspective on the issue. Describe the context in as much detail as needed.

   - Goal: The exercise aims to encourage students to look at similar situations and see different solutions and perspectives that may be formed from another student's cultural background.

   - Example: Two students with different backgrounds independently determine how they will address and resolve the moral dilemma.

2. **A moment in my shoes:** Select and describe a disability, then encourage students to navigate the local campus and/or community.

   - Goal: Promote understanding, allyship, inclusion, and belonging.

   - Example: Two students select a mobility device (i.e. walker, wheelchair, crutches), perform functional mobility, and assess accessibility while the other supervises. (Students can switch roles and perform the exercise again.)

3. **Assess, diagnose, and act:** Describe a DEI+ relevant situation, and have students discuss how they would take action to deliver a solution relevant to the objectives of the chapter.

   - Goal: To enhance students' skills in taking tangible actions to promote or serve issues related to DEI+ in their fieldwork and fieldwork education.

   - Example: As a class, discuss a scenario relevant to the topic, and come up with three viable solutions for action.

Bias and Microaggression

1. **Role play:** Student A is working with a new classmate (Student B) in the muscle-testing lab. Student B starts the conversation by saying, "Oh, I am so glad it is you I am partnering with this time. I can't take it with the accent with Maria (Student C) anymore. I can barely understand what she is saying." Maria is a Latina woman who recently immigrated to the country to study occupational therapy.

   - Goal: To challenge the students to take a perspective that they agree or disagree with.

   - Task: Student A takes this conversation forward to agree or disagree with Student B. Student B explains their perspective. Student C responds to both students. Then, all students switch roles and share how it feels to be in each role.

2. **Debate team:** Race, ethnicity, ability status, and other aspects of diversity should be considered when evaluating student performance in OT education. For example, it is acceptable to offer testing accommodations to students with learning difficulties. It should also be acceptable to provide accommodations to other aspects of diversity that facilitate or hinder students learning (e.g. race or socioeconomic status). Some may argue that this is a good approach to addressing social determinants of learning and growth. Others may argue that this approach perpetuates stereotypes and bias.

   - Goal: To make an argument supporting your thoughts based on lived experiences, evidence, laws, and/or expert opinions.

   - Task: Read an article, seek opinions, or compose an argument to discuss the issue from different perspectives.

   - Tips: Consider issues related to racism, critical race theory, and DEI+ laws.

3. **Take action:** Ask students to identify three actions that can mitigate bias or microaggressions toward one marginalized community that they identify with, are passionate about, or would like to advocate for in the classroom or fieldwork.

- Goal: To enhance students' skills to take tangible actions to promote or serve issues related to DEI+ in their education and early clinical practice.

- Example: Collaborate with the student leadership group to ask for a prayer room, all-gender, and inclusive bathrooms, or other actions needed to serve that marginalized group.

Privilege and Critical Consciousness

1. **Role play:** The OTA/OT practitioner/student formulates interview questions they would ask their clients/patients within a fieldwork or clinical situation, while being cognizant of their own implicit bias and how it may impact the therapeutic rapport.

   - Task: Participants develop a question for each of the following terms as they relate to a client/patient interaction, and reflect on how their sense of privilege may or may not impact their clinical reasoning skills:

     ◎ Health insurance status of a client

     ◎ Housing status of a client

     ◎ English as the spoken language of a client

     ◎ Political affiliation of a client

     ◎ The education level of a client.

2. **Debate team:** Ask students to consider the United States and how sociopolitical climate impact health and wellbeing at the individual and community levels. Next they engage a colleague, professor, peer, or friend on the statements below and actively seek out opinions and differing perspectives, and reflect on the impact within occupational therapy.

   - "An occupational therapy practitioner's (OTP) political affiliation does impact the therapeutic rapport."

   - "Having more wealth and resources contributes to a privileged sense of access and quality of healthcare services."

3. **Take action:** Advocacy is more than words; it's seen and unseen actions. Students could contact the state's AOTA representative assembly person (RA representative) via email and advocate on a topic they feel passionate about within the occupational therapy profession that they believe will make a lasting positive change. They should include evidence-based research if applicable and garner support from instructors, colleagues, mentors, peers, and local/state/national elected representatives. If unsure of who their RA representatives are, students can ask their occupational therapy state associations.

Cultural Humility

1. **Role play:** Student A is invited to their classmate's home (Student B) for a special faith/cultural-based dinner (e.g. Passover, Diwali, Eid, Christmas, or other occasions). Student B's parent (Person C) welcomes Student A warmly to their home and starts explaining the traditions behind the dinner. Then they ask Student A how their family celebrates that occasion.

   - Goal: To share information about cultural aspects that may or may not be similar to a classmate or a friend.

   - Task: Student A responds to the question and highlights similarities and differences between traditions. Student B explains how they feel about inviting their classmate to their home and considers how it feels if Student A celebrates that occasion similarly or differently from them.

2. **Debate team:** Christmas is widely celebrated in the US and other countries. It is the main holiday in academic calendars for schools, colleges, and other commercial and industrial sectors. Students are granted time off during the Christmas break with no need to ask for excused absences, unlike other religious holidays (e.g. Jewish or Muslim holidays). Students are calling for [insert holiday title] holiday/observance to be recognized as a major holiday where everyone takes the time off of work or school. Some students argue that although the law protects students against faith-based discrimination, it is unfair for them to miss schoolwork to celebrate their faith-based or cultural traditions.

   - Goal: To make an argument supporting students' thoughts based on lived experiences, evidence, laws, and/or expert opinions.

   - Task: Read an article, then seek opinions, or compose an argument to discuss the issue from different perspectives.

   - Tip: Students should consider issues of faith-based practices relevant to them.

3. **Take action:** Ask students to plan an idea for an event that highlights a cultural practice across different areas of occupation, including leisure activities (e.g. holding a culturally diverse sports event), self-care activities (e.g.

clothing across various cultures), and social participation activities (e.g. culturally diverse wedding practices).

- Goal: To enhance students' ability to share culturally relevant information with others in the classroom and advocate for one's culture.

- Example: Collaborate with the student leadership group to ask for virtual or physical space to hold one of these activities or events (e.g. virtual cultural cooking).

Empathy and Professionalism

1. **Role play:** The OTA/OT practitioner/student categorizes each of the following statements as a moral, professional or ethical dilemma and reflects on how they would handle each hypothetical situation within a professional setting.

   - Patient to therapist: "I do not have enough money for a co-payment. Can the clinic make an exception for today, please?"

   - OTA/OT student: "I feel sorry for Ms. Jackson. She doesn't seem to be the same since her partner passed away and I'm sure she's very depressed."

   - OTA student to instructor: "I don't think it's very fair for students who have religious observances to get more time to complete their assignments compared to those who are not religious."

2. **Debate team:** Students debate the following statement with an instructor, colleague, peer, or friend and consider the perspectives of all stakeholders before formulating an argument/stance.

   - "OTA/OT professionals should use social media platforms to publicly voice their own political stances."

3. **Take action:** Advocacy is more than words; it's seen and unseen actions. Students could send an email to any AOTA Board Director on a topic related to professionalism and/or the greater inclusion of empathy within the profession, and advocate using evidenced-based resources on how they believe it should be actualized within the profession as an ongoing practice

Fieldwork and Capstone

1. **Role play:** Describe common OTA and OT fundamental skills (i.e. transfers, standard assessment, ADL tasks). Describe the context in as much detail as needed.

   - Goal: To encourage students to experience the fieldwork power shift.

   - Example: Include two students with different backgrounds; one plays the fieldwork educator supervising and providing feedback while the other plays the student performing the task. After the activity, have a debrief meeting discussing strengths and areas of consideration for improvement.

2. **Express yourself:** Students select a random relevant DEI+ advocacy issue that encourages them to inform themselves (using their preferred personal information-seeking method), gather opinions, and compose an argument to present to classmates.

   - Goal: To increase advocacy skills and facilitate public speaking skills, as they are critical in fieldwork.

   - Example: Include one relevant evidence-based support reference for the DEI+ advocacy issue the student will present and advocate their position for, to their classmates.

3. **Flip the script:** Describe a scenario where students must take a different position in a real-life, relevant, professional situation that would differ from the position they would normally take in personal matters.

   - Goal: To enhance students' understanding of differing views and increase their ability to handle fieldwork relevant to DEI+ situations in their fieldwork education and early clinical practice.

   - Example: Two students play differing roles, one serving as the supervising occupational therapist and one as an occupational therapy assistant. Then, the students flip positions.

Student to Clinician

1. **Role play:** Student A has just moved to a new state/location for family reasons. They are also a new occupational therapy practitioner starting a new job at an inpatient hospital setting. They find themselves overwhelmed by the structure of their team, which seems to be made up mainly of one racial and ethnic group that they do not identify with. Student A contemplates whether they will fit into the group given their intersectionality and their limited clinical experience and familiarity with the area. Another new therapist (Student B), who identifies with the same racial and ethnic group as Student A, approaches Student A and welcomes them to the team. Student A shares their excitement about starting the job but also their concerns about the team structure. A seasoned therapist who identifies with the majority group in the team (Person C) seems very friendly, and welcomes Student A to the team, asking them to reach out if they have any concerns about the new role.

   - Goal: To practice expressing concerns related to aspects of DEI+ for newly qualified practitioners.

   - Task: Student A starts the conversation with Student B and states their thoughts and feelings about the team structure. Student B shares some advice from what they have learned over their short time in the team. Person C shares what they perceive about Student A and what would make them succeed on the team despite the intersectional differences.

2. **Debate team:** Debate this statement: "Diversity hires are both fair and biased" (i.e. the perception that someone was hired to fill an expected number of positions meant to diversify the workplace, or people with DEI+ attributes such as a Black therapist are hired to diversify the racial profile of staff).

   - Goal: To prompt students to make an argument supporting their thoughts based on lived experiences, evidence, laws, and/or expert opinions.

   - Task: Read an article, seek opinions, or compose an argument to discuss the statement from different perspectives.

3. **Take action:** Plan an in-service training on culturally relevant clinical practices. Use your intersectionality, culture, faith, race, ethnicity, and ability status for the first in-service session. Provide relevant and accurate examples

of daily activities related to that group including considerations for the OT process (e.g. assessment tools to consider, interventions).

- Goal: To enhance students' ability to promote and recognize culturally relevant information with team members in the workplace.

Index

Page references to Figures have the letter f following the page number, while references to Tables are followed by t

AAA (allyship, accompliceship
    and advocacy) 29–43
    action-oriented thinking 42
    case example 30
    critic al thinking 42
    and fieldwork 30, 40–1
        intricate components of student
            experience 29–30
    reasons for importance 31–2
    reflective thinking 42
    terminology 33–4t
    worksheet 159
AAPI-OT *see* Association of Asian
    Americans and Pacific Islanders in
    Occupational Therapy (AAPI-OT)
AAVE *see* African American
    Vernacular English (AAVE)
ableism 71, 84, 97, 139
academic fieldwork coordinators
    (AFWCs) 113–14, 115, 119, 124, 125
academic work versus personal
    well-being 32
accompliceship
    as an action, not an identity 32
    case examples 30
    clinician, becoming 139
    commitment and action, involving
        36–7
    defining 36
    terminology 33–4t
accountability 70–2, 100, 107
    and empathy 94, 101–6, 143
Accreditation Council for Occupational
    Education (ACOTE®) Standards 115

action-oriented thinking 157
allyship, accompliceship and
    advocacy 32, 36–7, 42
bias, intersectionality and
    microaggressions 59, 160
clinician, becoming 145, 167–8
critical consciousness 75
cultural humility 91, 163–4
DEI+ 27, 158
empathy and professionalism 108, 165
fieldwork and capstone 126
next generation of OT students
    and DEI+ 145
privilege and critical
    consciousness 75, 162
active engagement 103
activities of daily living (ADLs) 124
advocacy 38–9
    case examples 39
    clinician, becoming 139
    defining 38
    effective 38
    enhancing sense of 38–9
    forms 38
    and harm done to classmates of color 52
    in OT education 23–4
    and student DEI+ 23–4
    terminology 33–4t
African American community 52
African American Vernacular
    English (AAVE) 52
AFWCs *see* academic fieldwork
    coordinators (AFWCs)
alliances 34–5

allyship 34–5, 36
as an action, not an identity 32
case examples 30, 35–6
clinician, becoming 139
defining 34
and harm done to classmates of color 52
learning 34
and peer-mentorship 143
terminology 33–4t
see also AAA (allyship, accompliceship and advocacy); alliances
American Hospital Association 112
American Occupational Therapy Association (AOTA) 16, 68, 131
Assembly of Student Delegates 40
Boardroom to Classroom program 39–40
ethical code 16–17, 132
and bias 56, 57
and empathy 93, 96, 101, 106, 107
analytics 102
anatomy 31
Angelou, Maya 95
AOTA *see* American Occupational Therapy Association (AOTA)
Arab American Occupational Therapy Group 35
Association of Asian Americans and Pacific Islanders in Occupational Therapy (AAPI-OT) 35
audience engagement 102
audio-visual multimedia 101

bias
action-oriented thinking 59
case examples 45, 51–2
critical thinking 59
defining 46
and difficult conversations in the classroom 50–2
disturbances instigated by 84
explicit 19t, 24–5, 44, 48t
gender-specific 58
identifying and articulating 34, 47, 53
implicit 17, 19t, 24–5, 65–6, 70, 97, 157, 162
and microaggressions 44, 46, 48t, 54, 58
incidents of, recognizing 54
and intersectionality 53–7
action-oriented thinking 59
case example 56–7
in the classroom 53–4

critical thinking 59
reflective thinking 59
in lecture content 50
Macro-Micro Model of Diversity (MMMD) 54–5
microaggressions as projections of personal biases 47
normalizing 47
personal 56
and power 47, 53–4
preconceived knowledge contributing to 53
and privilege 53–4
recognizing 46–7, 53, 54
reflective thinking 59
terminology related to 48t
types 47
worksheet 160–1
see also microaggressions
Black Americans/Canadians 52
brand management 102
BroOT movement 35
Brothas advocacy group 35

capstone educators 114
Castro, D. 79
CC *see* critical consciousness (CC)
Chomsky, Noam 63
clinical empathy 97–8
strategies for employing 98–9t
clinical learning 64, 65, 70
DEI+ in 24–5
clinical simulations 101
clinician, becoming 128–46
action-oriented thinking 145
case examples 131, 132, 135–6, 137–8
from classroom to the clinic 130–2
critical thinking 145
cultural changes 138–40
first year as an OT practitioner 137–8
professional development, engagement and DEI 134–5
reflective thinking 144
seeing the larger picture 133–4
transition versus transformation 132–3
worksheet 167–8
Coalition of Occupational Therapy Advocates for Diversity (COTAD) 14, 37, 131
codes of conduct/ethics 36, 56, 132
empathy 93, 96, 101, 106–8

see also American Occupational
  Therapy Association (AOTA)
Coin Model of Privilege and
  Critical Allyship 71
collaboration 38, 103, 105, 119, 134, 144
  interprofessional 53, 68
  and participation 105
communities of practice 137
community 63, 84, 134, 143
  Black/African American 125
  building 141
  caring 137
  and cultural humility 83–5
  engagement with 78, 83–5
  health promotion 68
  health settings 120
  Hispanic/Latino/LatinX 91
  and the individual 84
  initiatives 141
  interventions, community-based 82
  LGBTQIA+ 56
  and Macro-Micro Model of Diversity 54
  marginalized 82, 90
  members from diverse backgrounds 142
  organizations 139
  OT 133, 143
  outreach programs 139
  partners 124
  religious holidays, importance to 83
  sense of 62, 142
  sharing feelings of 97
community-based events 135
community-based organizations 134
community-based programs 140
community-based projects 144
community-based supporters
  and advocates 135
community-centered practices 129
community-dwelling persons 84
constructive feedback 32
content 10, 23, 51
  clinical 133
  creation of 102
  curating of 103
  digital 104
  generation of 105, 106t
  interpretation of 105, 106t
  lectures 50
  triggering 11
continuous learning 102, 105

copyright 104
COTAD *see* Coalition of Occupational
  Therapy Advocates for
  Diversity (COTAD)
crisis management 102
critical consciousness (CC)
  action-oriented thinking 75
  addressing SDOH 67
  case examples 69–70, 72–4
  critical thinking 74
  cultural competence, promoting 66
  defining/meaning for students
    and practitioners 64–70
  empowering those served 66–7
  future challenges, preparing for 68–9
  health equity, fostering 67
  healthcare delivery, improving 68
  implicit biases, recognizing 65–6
  interprofessional collaboration,
    enhancing 68
  and marginalized groups 64–6
  reflective thinking 74
  social justice, advancing 67–8
  structural inequities, understanding 65
  see also privilege
critical thinking
  allyship, accompliceship and advocacy 42
  clinician, becoming 145
  critical consciousness 74
  cultural humility 91
  DEI+ 27, 105
  empathy and professionalism 108
  fieldwork and capstone 126
  intersectionality 59
  next generation of OT students
    and DEI+ 145
  privilege 74
cultural competence 66, 80
cultural humility 19t, 77–92
  action-oriented thinking 91
  case examples 82–3, 84–5, 86–7, 88–91
  in the classroom 21–2, 82–3
  in clinical practice 85–6
  critical thinking 91
  and DEI+ 21–3
  in fieldwork education 85–6
  harmful effects of OT practices lacking 77
  as an intentional mindset needed for
    ethical and inclusive practices 77
  and intersectionality 87–90

cultural humility *cont.*
  as a mindset 79, 80, 82
  and power 21, 78, 82, 87
  and privilege 87–90
  productive approach to 90
  reflective thinking 91
  related terminology 80, 81*t*
  and similar terms 80
  in social and healthcare sciences 80
  terminology 80, 81*t*
  worksheet 163–4
culture 16, 53, 121, 167
  Black 19–20
  change 129, 138–40
  cinematic 71
  culture-centered terms 80
  and disability 79
  diversity within 83
  dynamic nature of 80
  education 133
  and food 22
  of inclusion 142
  knowledge gaps 21
  and Macro-Micro Model of
    Diversity 54, 55*f*, 57
  and privilege 61
  recognizing one's own 82
  role in daily functioning 113
  work 130
cybersecurity awareness 104

DCC *see* doctoral capstone
    coordinator (DCC)
debate teams 157
  bias and microaggressions 160
  clinician, becoming 167
  cultural humility 163
  DEI+ 158
  empathy and professionalism 165
  privilege and critical consciousness 162
DEI+ (Diversity, Equity, Inclusion, and Other
    Aspects of Social Justice) 13–27
  action-oriented thinking 27
  advocacy and self-advocacy 40
  basic terminology 18–19*t*
  being DEI+ mindful practitioner
    78, 128, 132, 133, 136
  case example 14, 15
  in clinical and fieldwork learning 24–5
  critical thinking 27

  and cultural humility 21–3
  and empathy 94, 97
  in fieldwork 24–5, 118–20
  lack of 110
  and next generation of OT students 141–3
  polarization of 112
  professional development and
    engagement 134–5
  reasons for learning about 16–20
  reflective thinking 27
  student DEI+ and advocacy
    in education 23–4
  student diversity 19–20
  underrepresentation 15–16
  workbook, exercises and discussion
    prompts 156–68
  worksheet 158
  see also AAA (allyship, accompliceship
    and advocacy); accompliceship;
    advocacy; allyship
digital citizenship 104–6
digital footprint management 104
digital inclusion, promoting 105
digital literacy 104
digital technologies, integration within
    health science education 101
dignity, core value of 36
disabled people, bias against 46
  Black women with disabilities 57, 58
  and culture 79
  invisible disabilities 78
discrimination 20, 139
  explicit 88
  faith-based/religious 163
  by fieldwork supervisors 26
  healthcare systems, within 67
  and heterosexism 71
  incidents of 53, 138
  learning environments 30, 45, 111
  racial 26
  witnessing 54
  working environments 129
DiverseOT (advocacy group) 37
Diversity, Equity, Inclusion, and Other
    Aspects of Social Justice *see* DEI+
    (Diversity, Equity, Inclusion, and
    Other Aspects of Social Justice)
doctor of occupational therapy (OTD) 10, 14
doctoral capstone coordinator (DCC) 115–16
dress codes 37–8

empathy 93–109
  absence of 96
  and accountability 94, 101–6, 143
  action-oriented thinking 108
  case examples 99–100, 106–7
  clinical 97–9
  components of 93
  critical thinking 108
  and DEI+ 94, 97
  and fostering a deep therapeutic
      relationship 95
  and professionalism 101
  reflective thinking 108
  strategies for employing clinical
      empathy 98–9t
  versus sympathy 96, 97, 98
  traditional 98
  value within healthcare education 96
  worksheet 165
empowerment 66–7
e-professionalism 62, 101
ethical considerations 102
ethics
  AOTA code 16–17, 132
    and bias 56, 57
    and empathy 93, 96, 101, 106, 107
  behavior 103, 104, 107
  case examples 35
  client-centered care 46
  and cultural humility 77
  decision-making 113
  ethical and moral conflicts 62
  ethical DEI+ mindful practitioner 128,
      132
  ethical dilemmas 107, 165
  ethical violations 36, 41, 107, 108
  guidelines 103
  online behavior 104
  and privilege 70–3
  professional 124, 132
  prudence, principle of 120
  social media engagement 105
  standards 100, 102, 138
  therapeutic relationship 79
explicit bias 19t, 24–5, 44, 48t

faith groups 135–6
feedback 26, 46
  case examples 87, 119–23, 125
  constructive 32, 104

critical 113, 120
  on DEI+ content 23
  negative 102
  objective 120
  peer-reviewed 144
  on performance 86
  presentation delivery 51
  on professional behaviors 51
  role play 166
  seeking 103–4
  student 120
  when provided 114
fidelity, principle of 36
fieldwork and capstone 110–27
  AAA on 40–1
  academic fieldwork coordinators 113–14
  action-oriented thinking 126
  case examples 40–1, 119–20, 122–3
  coordinators and education,
      case example 122–3
  critical thinking 126
  cultural humility in fieldwork
      education 85
  de-escalation in 120–2
  and DEI+ 24–5, 118–20
  difficult conversations in the
      classroom 124–5
  education 110, 124–5
  journey, experience and entry
      into the profession 112
  Level I and Level II placements 40,
      113, 114, 119, 124, 125, 131
  navigating tough situations 120–2
  self-advocacy 40
  terms and roles related to education in
      occupational therapy 116–18t
  worksheet 166
fieldwork educators (FWEs) 114
freedom of speech, concept of 107
Freire, P. 65
future challenges, preparing for 68–9
FWE (OT fieldwork educator) 86, 87

grade point average (GPA) 32

hate crimes 84, 123
health equity, fostering 67
healthcare delivery, improving 68
healthcare practitioners 46, 107
heterosexism, as dominant norm 71

implicit biases 17, 19*t*, 24–5,
    70, 79, 97, 157, 162
  bias and microaggressions 44,
    46, 48*t*, 54, 58
  in healthcare practitioners 46
  recognizing 65–6
  and stereotypes 25
imposter syndrome 140
inequality, systems of 71
intellectual property 104
interprofessional collaboration,
    enhancing 68
intersectionality
  action-oriented thinking 59
  and bias 53–7
    action-oriented thinking 59
    in the classroom 53–4
    critical thinking 59
    reflective thinking 59
  case example 45
  critical thinking 59
  and cultural humility 87–90
  defining 53
  intersectionality wheel 58*f*
  map 55*f*
  and privilege 87–90
  recognizing 54
  reflective thinking 59
  wheel 57, 58*f*
introduction to OT 31
Islamophobia 123

kinesiology 31

Langston Hughes, James Mercer 31
liberation 37
life events 55

Macro-Micro Model of Diversity
    (MMMD) 54–5, 57
marginalized communities/
    groups 15, 26, 71, 82, 139
  and accomplices 37
  and allyship 34–5
  and critical consciousness 64–6
  identifying with 53
  implicit biases, recognizing 65
  limited exposure to 90
  and MDI networks 35
  and microaggressions 47

Master of Science in Occupational
    Therapy (MSOT) 14, 41
MDI (multicultural, diversity, and
    inclusion) networks 35
media literacy 105
microaggressions 48–50, 73, 97
  active and passive forms 44
  behaviors 47
  case examples 45, 48–52
  defining 47
  in didactic or clinical education 47
  forms 44, 47
  in occupational therapy education
    49–50
  as projections of personal biases 47
  stereotypes, perpetuating 47
  terminology related to 48*t*
  worksheet 160–1
  see also bias
MMMD *see* Macro-Micro Model
    of Diversity (MMMD)
MSOT *see* Master of Science in
    Occupational Therapy (MSOT)
multicultural, diversity, and inclusion
    networks *see* MDI (multicultural,
    diversity, and inclusion) networks
multi-faith panels 135–6

National Black Occupational Therapy
    Caucus Network for LGBTQIA+
    Concerns in Occupational Therapy 35
National Board for Certification in
    Occupational Therapy (NBCOT) 131
Network of Occupational Therapy
    Practitioners with Disabilities
    and Supporters (NOTPD) 35

Obama, Barack 46
occupational therapy assistant
    (OTA) 10, 30, 32, 40
  Occupational Therapy for Native
    Americans (OTNA) 35
occupational therapy (OT) 30, 32
  advocacy in education 23–4, 40
  first semester 30, 31
  and human diversity 86
  next generation of OT students
    and DEI+ 141–5
  terms and roles related to
    education in 116–18*t*

occupational therapy practitioners
(OTPs) 16, 17, 79, 96
  bias and intersectionality 53
  DEI+ mindful practitioners 133
  empathy 96
  fieldwork 125
  first year 129, 136–8
  inclusive environments, creating 142
  self-advocacy 40
  solutions, finding 121
  working with individuals of
      different backgrounds 132
  see also occupational therapy assistant
      (OTA); occupational therapy (OT)
OJOTC see Orthodox Jewish Occupational
  Therapy Chavrusa (OJOTC)
older people, bias against 46
online behavior 104
oppression 44, 53, 67
  dismantling systems of 34, 36, 91
  perceived sense of 74
  suffered by women 88
Orthodox Jewish Occupational Therapy
  Chavrusa (OJOTC) 35
OT see occupational therapy (OT)
OTA see occupational therapy
  assistant (OTA)
OTD see doctor of occupational therapy (OTD)
OTNA see Occupational Therapy for
  Native Americans (OTNA)
overweight people, bias against 46

participation 105
peer-mentorship 143
personal information, protecting 104
power
  and bias 47, 53–4
  case example 87
  challenging of power structures 36
  components of 80
  controlling of a student's performance
      evaluation/passing grade 87
  and cultural humility 21, 78, 82, 87
  defining 79
  DEI+ and cultural humility 21
  healthcare systems, within 67
  and privilege 53–4, 62, 79–80, 82
  and social privilege 88
  of student-led organization in
      student advocacy 24

  of supervisor 87
  in a therapeutic relationship 79
privilege
  action-oriented thinking 75
  awareness of 61
  and bias 44, 53–4
  confronting injustice and oppression 36
  confronting one's own 34
  continuum of 82
  critical thinking 74
  and cultural humility 87–90
  and culture 61
  defining 61
  demographic and social
      characteristics 72t
  direct and direct sense of 62
  factors related to 62
  and intersectionality 87–90
  as a multifaceted construct 61–2
  and power 53–4, 62, 79–80, 82
  recognizing related factors 70–2
  reflective thinking 74
  sense of 72t
  social 82
  as a social determinant of health 62
  whether accountability and ethics
      are included 70–2
  worksheet 162
  see also critical consciousness
professionalism 62, 94, 96, 108, 114
  creating professional profiles 103
  and empathy 100, 101, 165
  examples of professional engagement
      opportunities 128
  professional development 134–5
  professional identity 139–40
  worksheet 165

racism 67, 70, 71, 139, 160
  by fieldwork educator 40–1
  stereotypes 41
  systemic 59, 124
rapport 32, 50, 66, 142
  therapeutic 70, 96, 162
reflective thinking
  allyship, accompliceship and advocacy 42
  bias and intersectionality 59
  clinician, becoming 144
  critical consciousness 74
  cultural humility 91

reflective thinking *cont.*
  DEI+ 27
  empathy and professionalism 108
  fieldwork and capstone 126
  next generation of OT students
    and DEI+ 144
  privilege 74
risk-taking, accompliceship 36
role play 10, 156–7, 166
  allyship, accompliceship and
    advocacy 159
  bias and microaggressions 160
  clinician, becoming 167
  cultural humility 163
  DEI+ 158
  empathy and professionalism 165
  fieldwork and capstone 166
  privilege and critical consciousness 162

SDOH (social determinants of health),
  addressing 63, 64, 67, 84
search engines 101
self-advocacy 40, 68, 107
sexual orientation 71
social determinants of health (SDOH)
  see SDOH (social determinants
  of health), addressing
social justice, advancing 67–8
social media competency 101, 102–4, 105
social media platforms 100
  active engagement on 103
  case example 106, 107
  content creation 102
  crisis management 102
  familiarity with 102
  features and functionalities 101
  following relevant accounts on 102
  personal 100
  public 100
  Social Media Competency Scale 106*t*
  strategic networking 103
  using to voice political stances 165
social systems 54
SOTA *see* Student Organization for
  Occupational Therapy (SOTA)

state board elections 140
staying informed 103
stereotypes 70, 157
  and implicit bias 25
  perpetuating 47, 160
  racist 41
strategic networking 103
structural inequities, understanding 65
Student Organization for Occupational
  Therapy (SOTA) 31, 37
support systems 32, 142
  professional 125
  social 64
  supplemental 122
sympathy, versus empathy 96, 97, 98

TODOS (Terapia Ocupacional para
  Diversidad, Oportunidad,
  y Solidaridad), network of
  Hispanic practitioners 35
Tubman, Harriet 130

unspoken rules, as barriers 38

Villarosa, L. 15
virtual software, simulated 69

Web 2.0 technology 101
webinars 103
women
  Afro-Latina 85
  Black women with disabilities 57, 58
  gender-specific biases affecting 58
  injustices and oppression suffered by
    88
  lived experiences of 85
  of marginalized communities 84
  privileged 84
  transgender 84
workshops, attending 103
World Health Organization (WHO) 63
Wright Edelman, Marian 112

Zhu, S. 105